COW COLORING BOOK

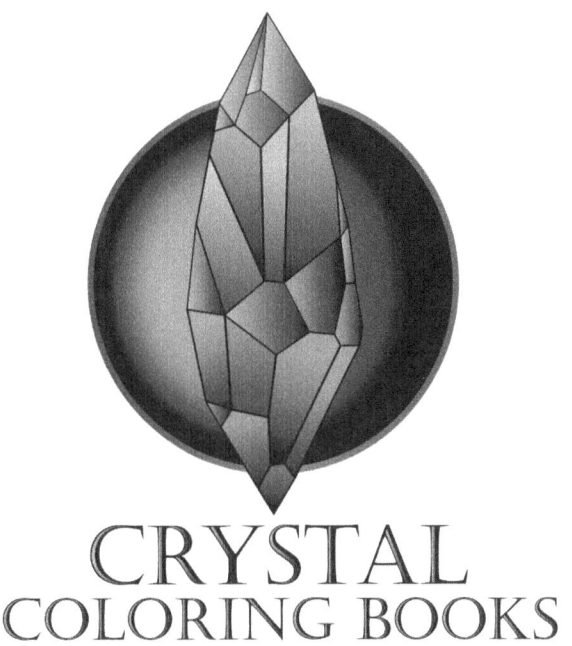

CRYSTAL COLORING BOOKS

Copyright © 2017 Crystal Coloring Books
All rights reserved.

ISBN-13: 978-1986055642
ISBN-10: 1986055647

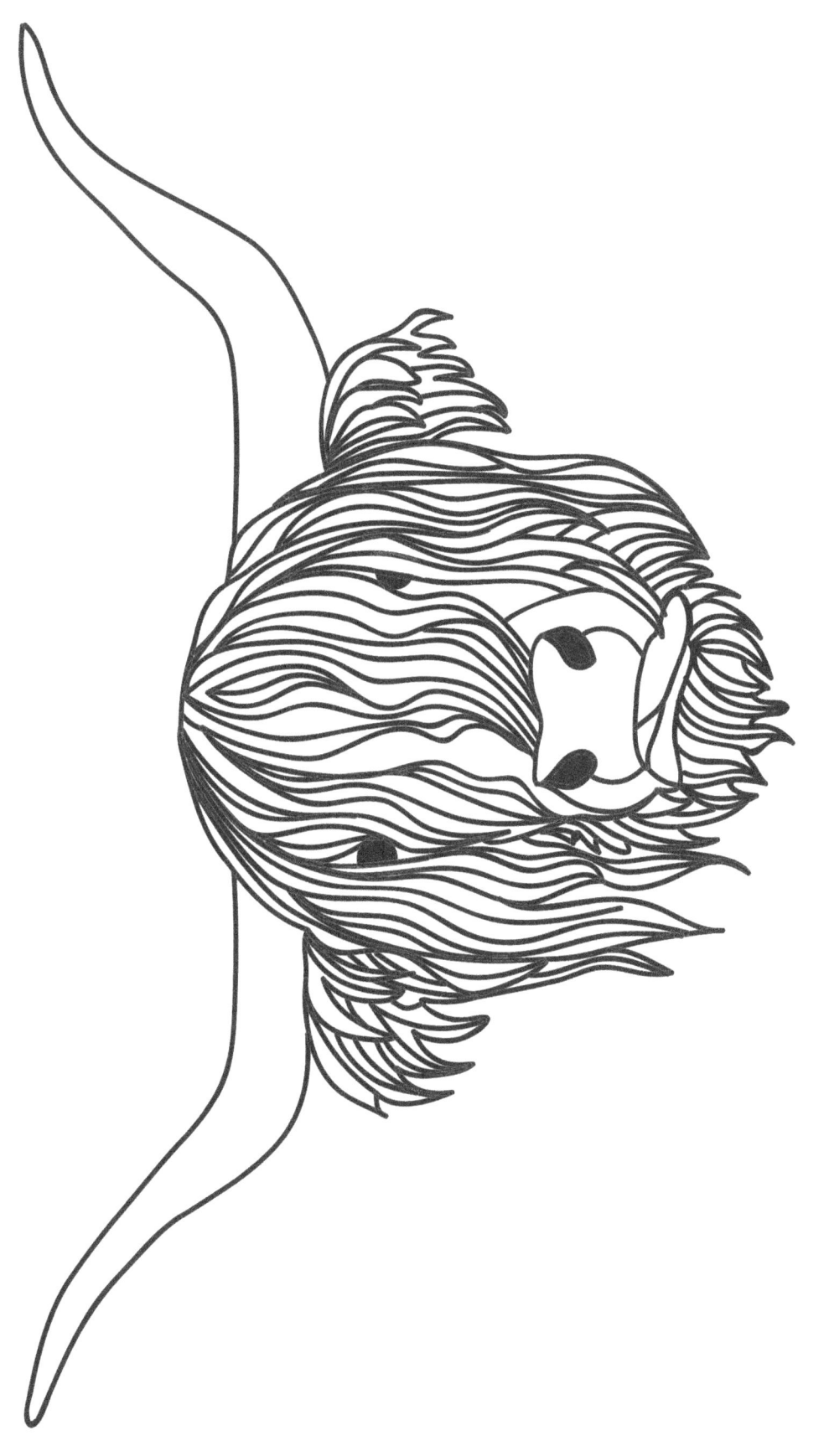

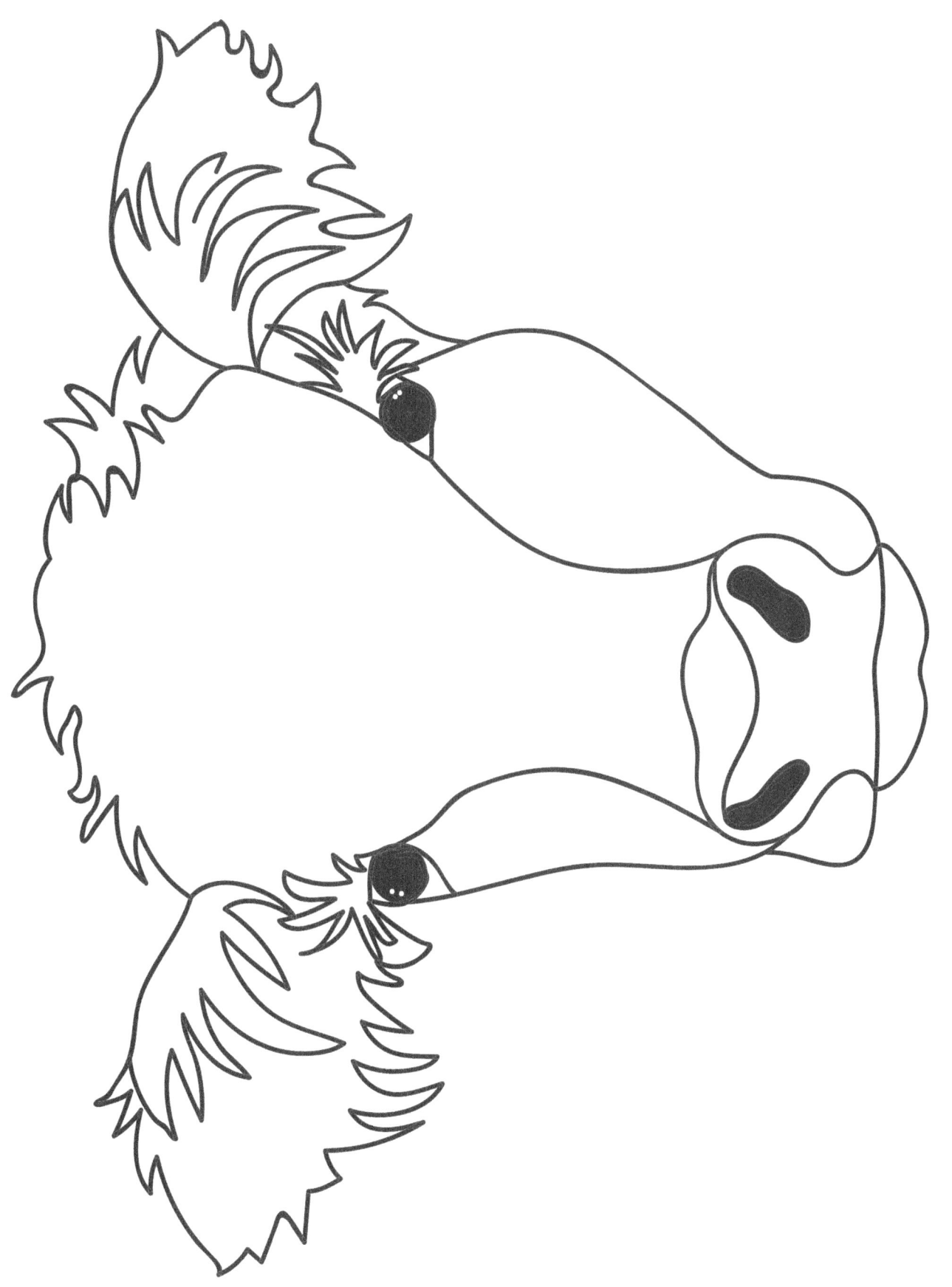

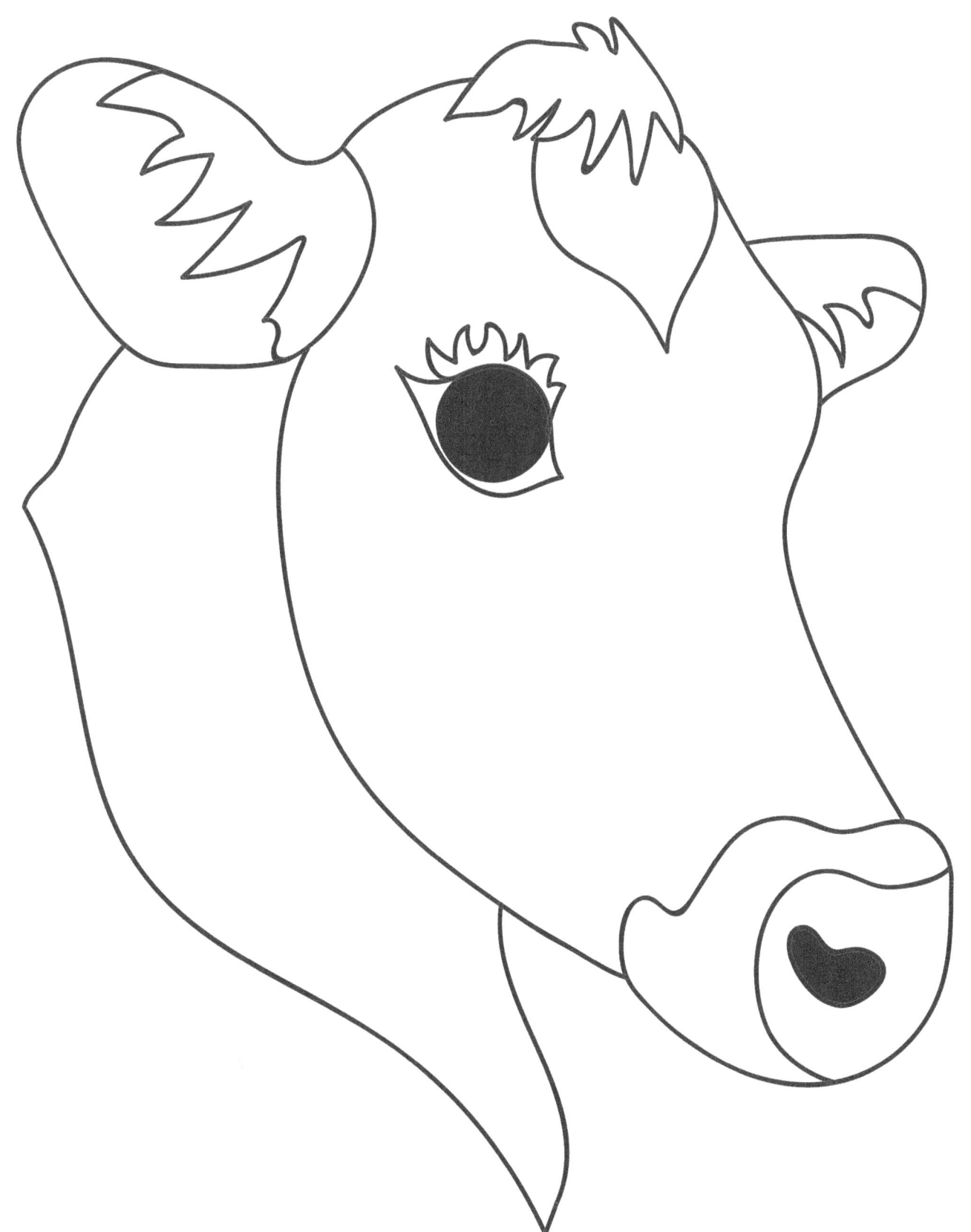

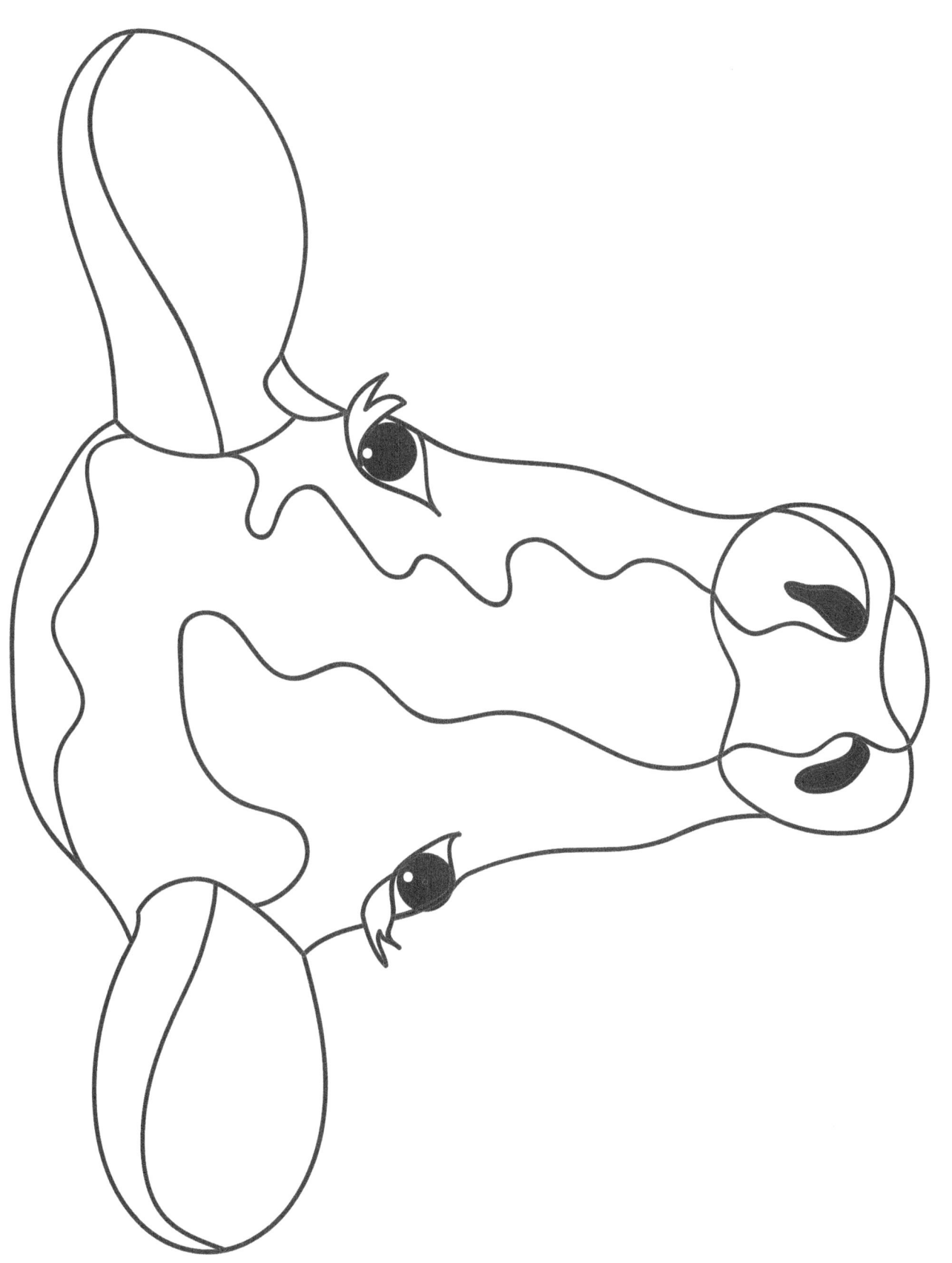

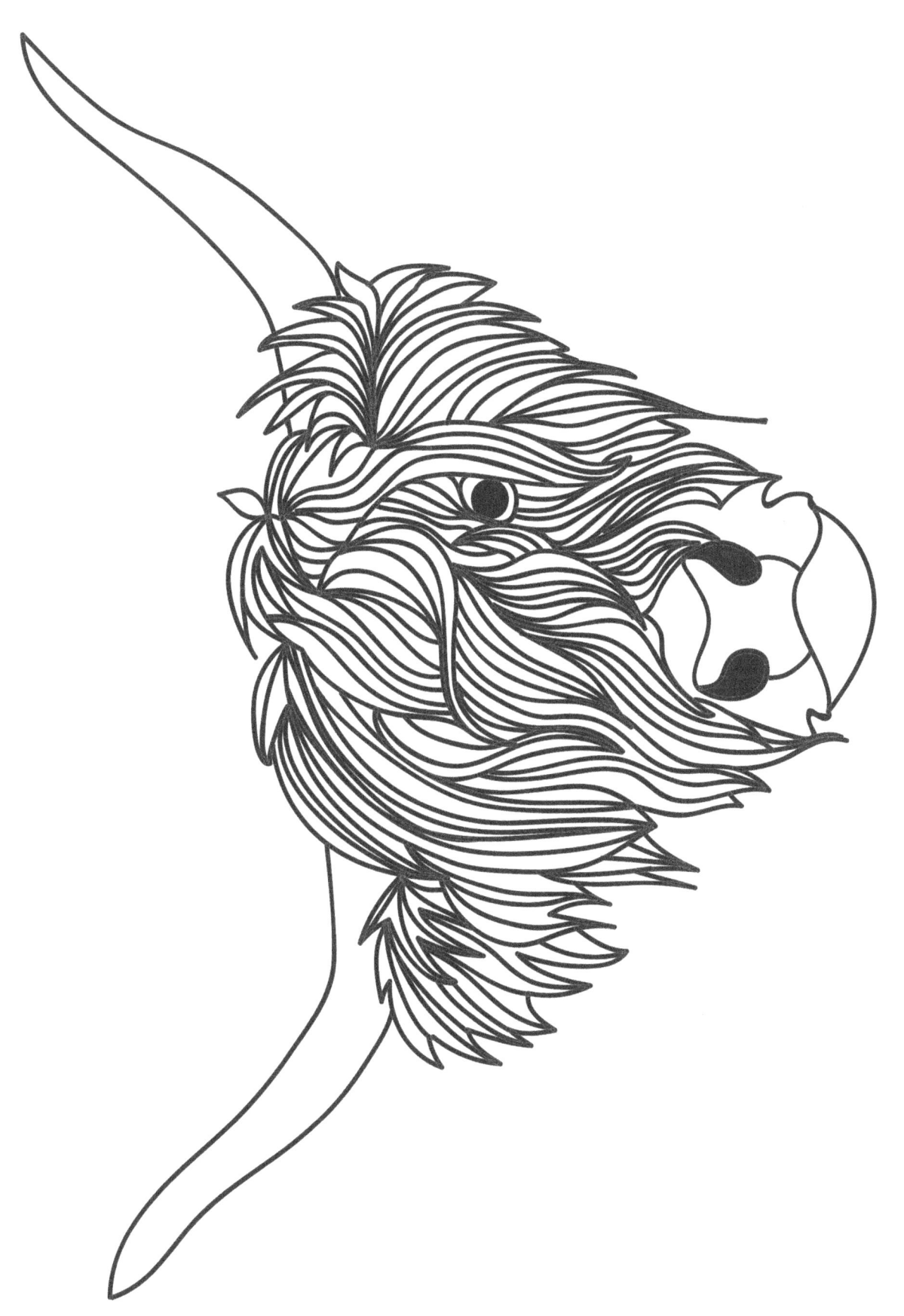

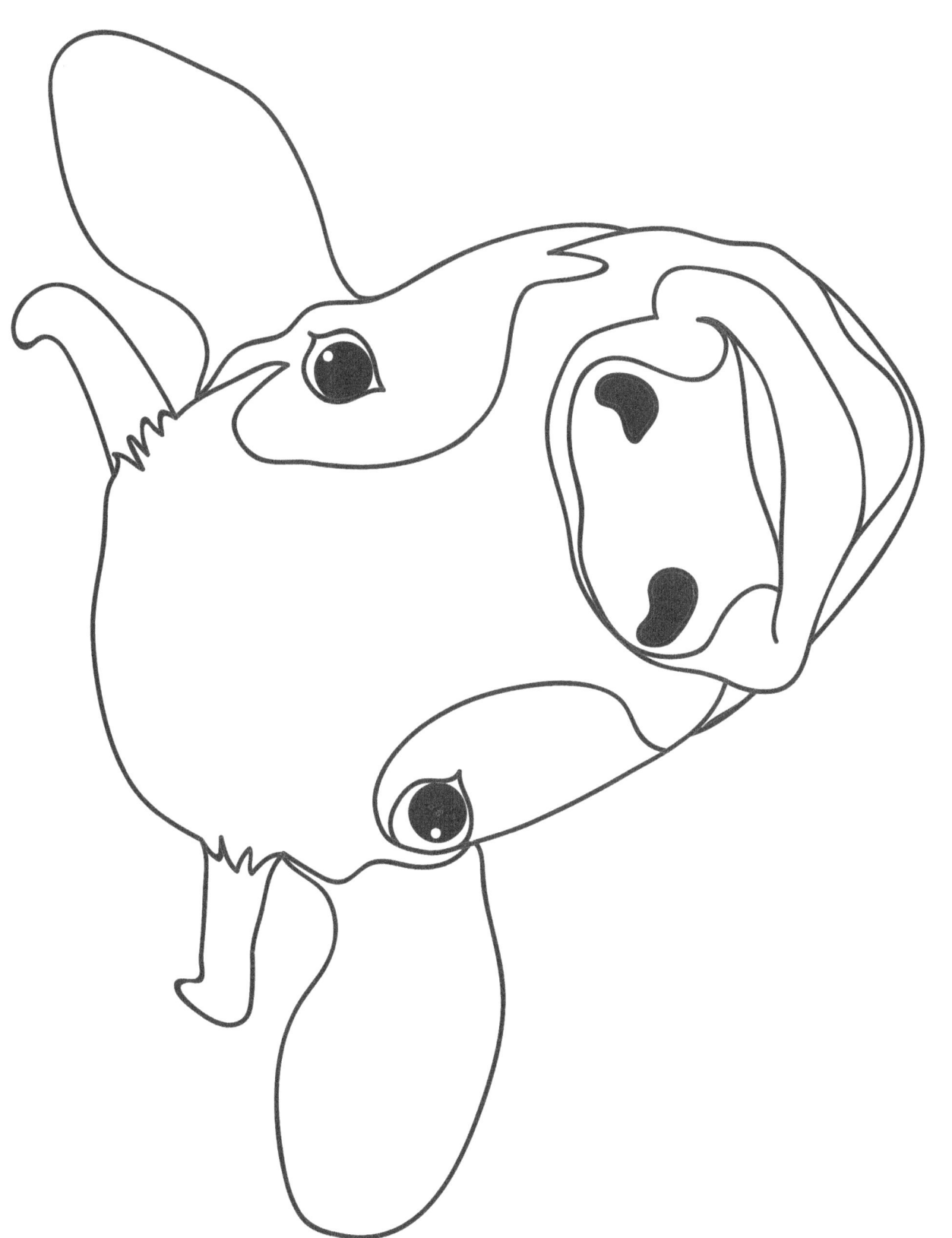

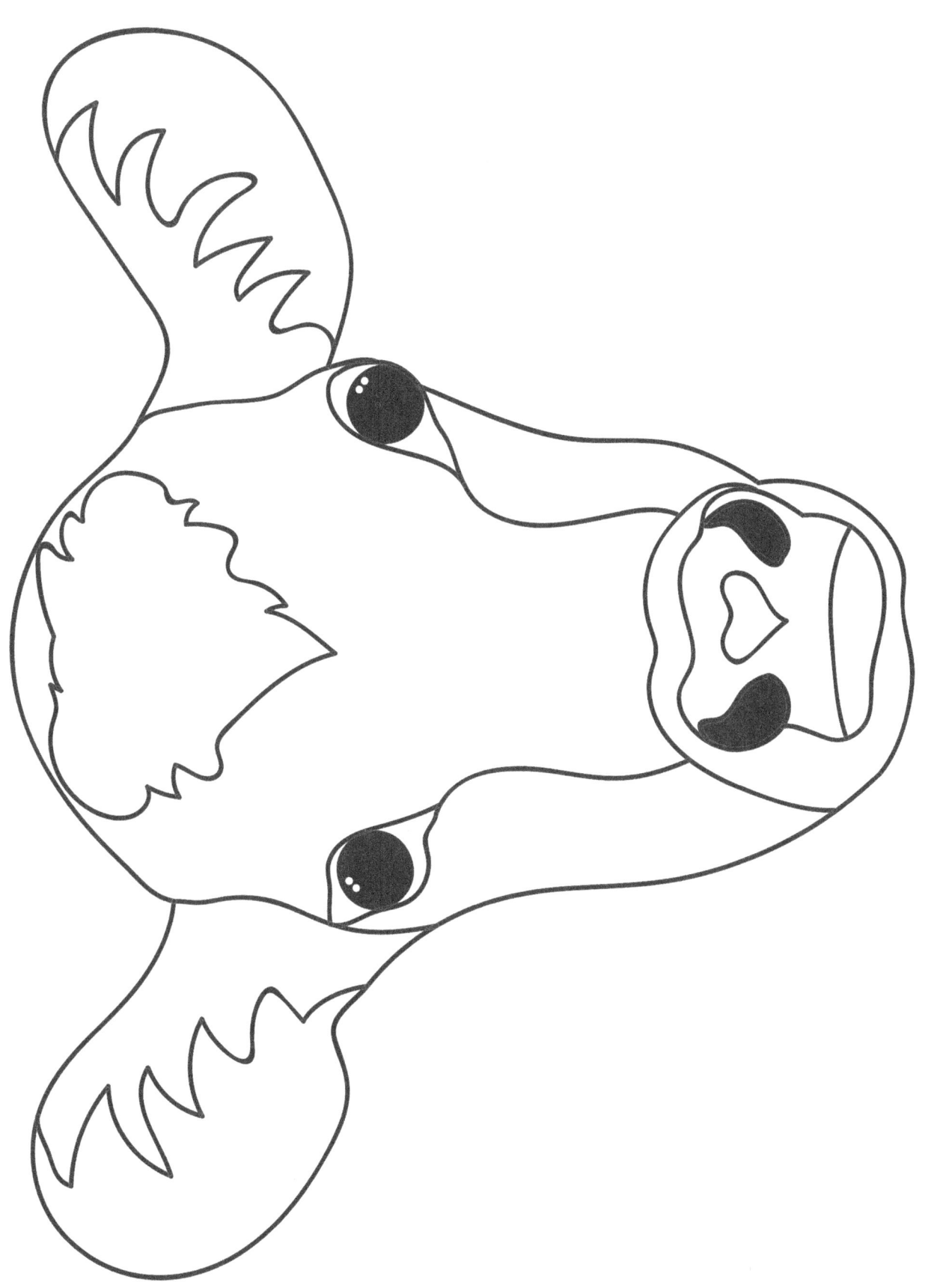

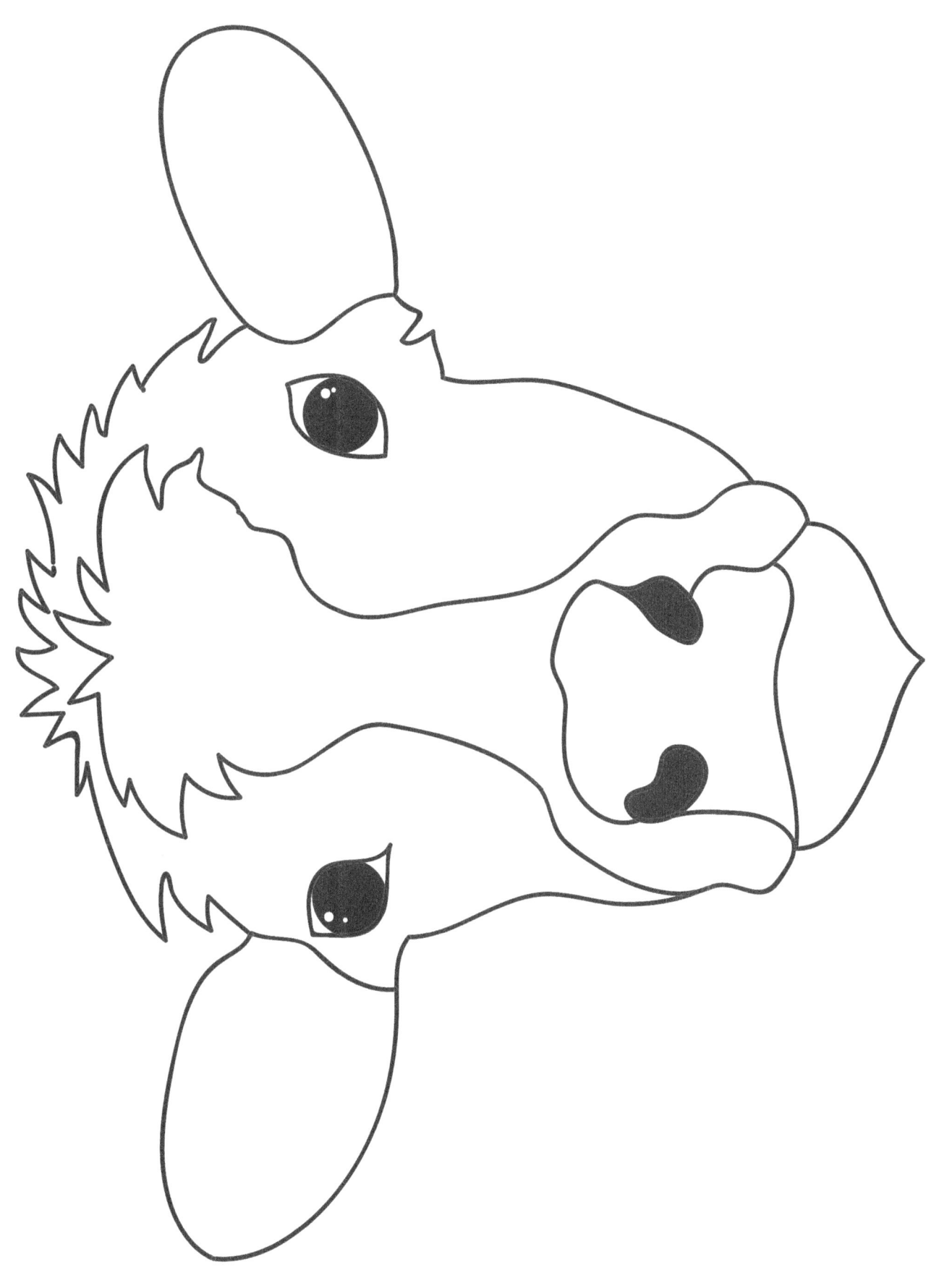

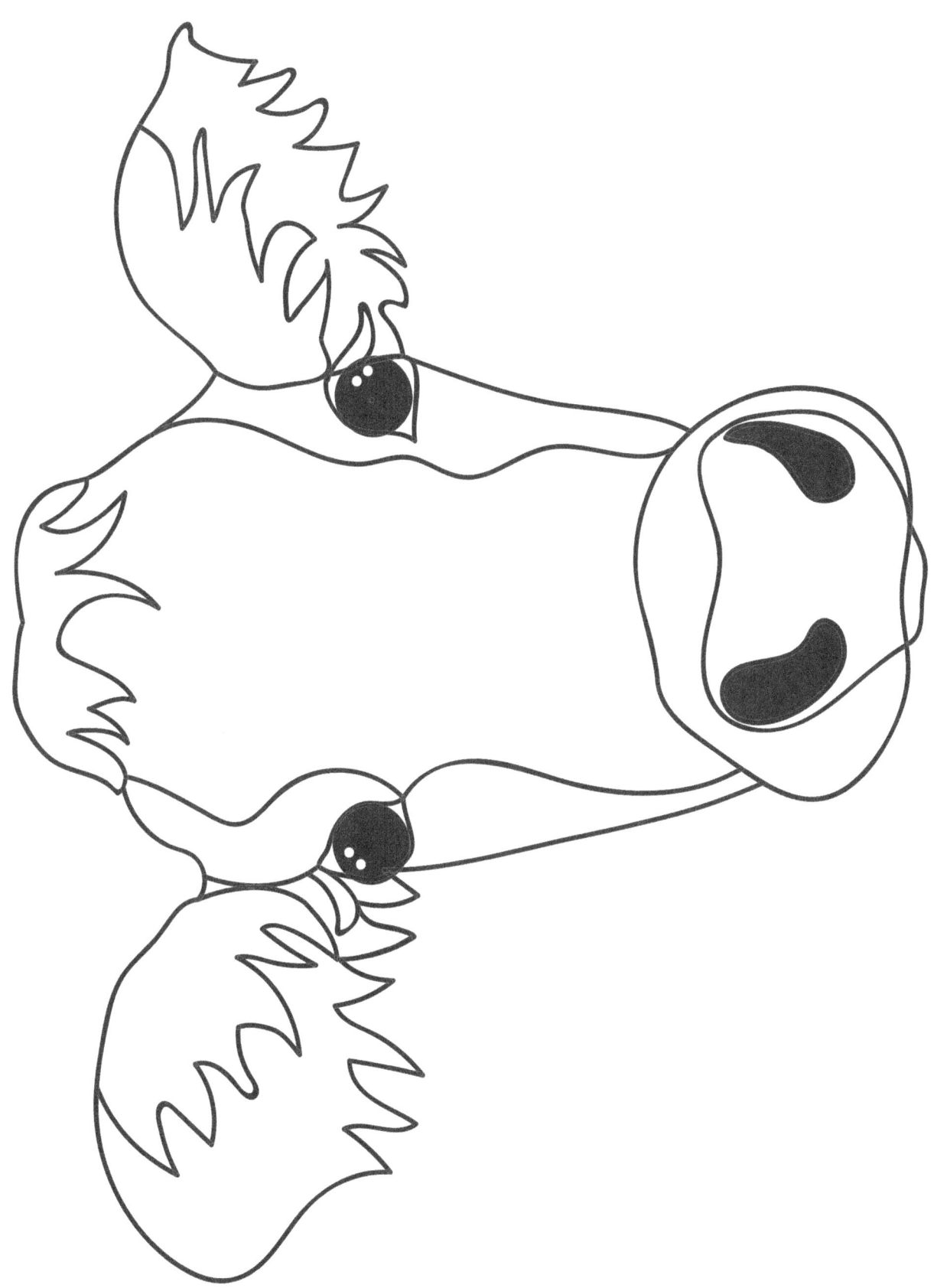

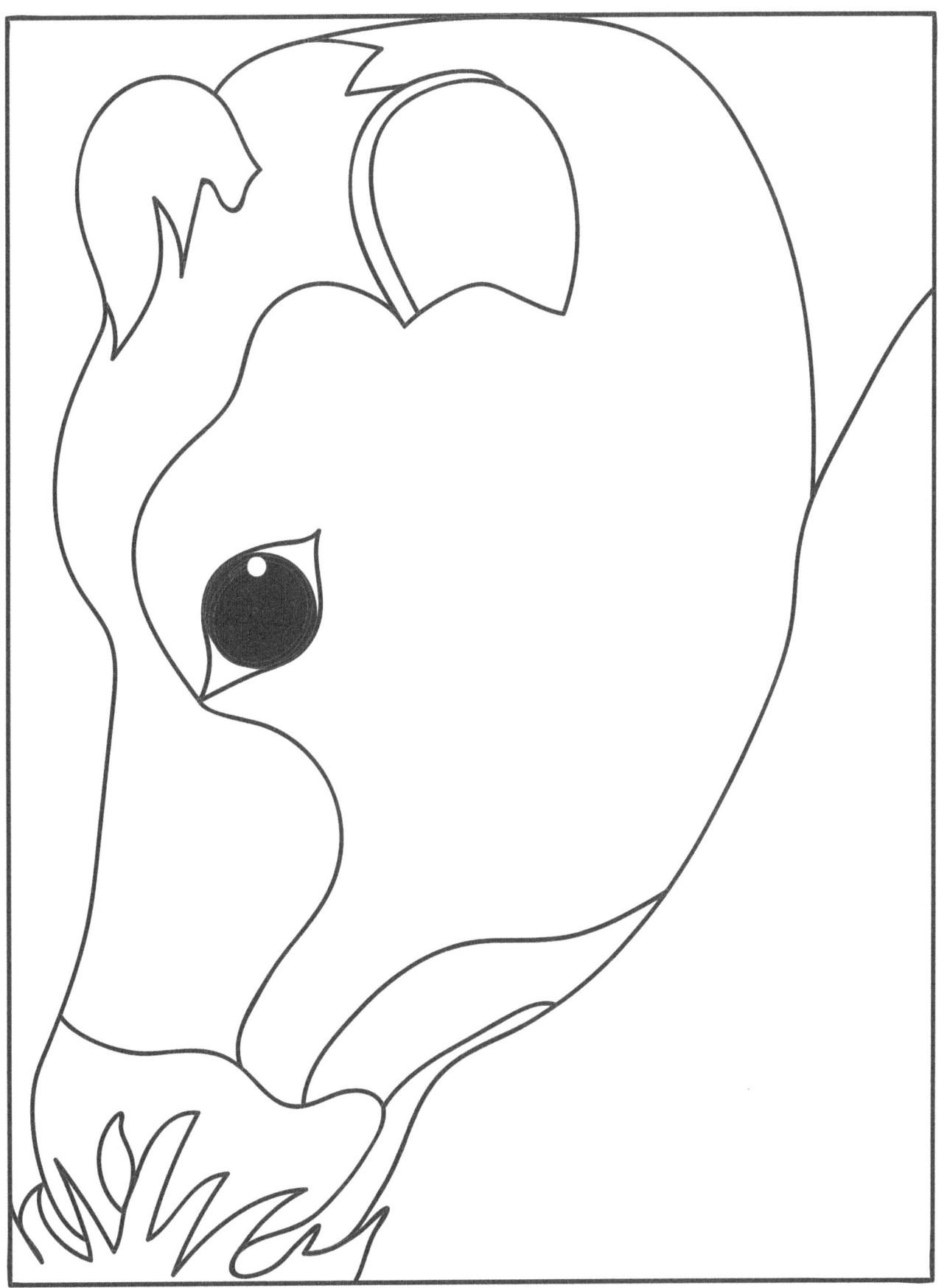

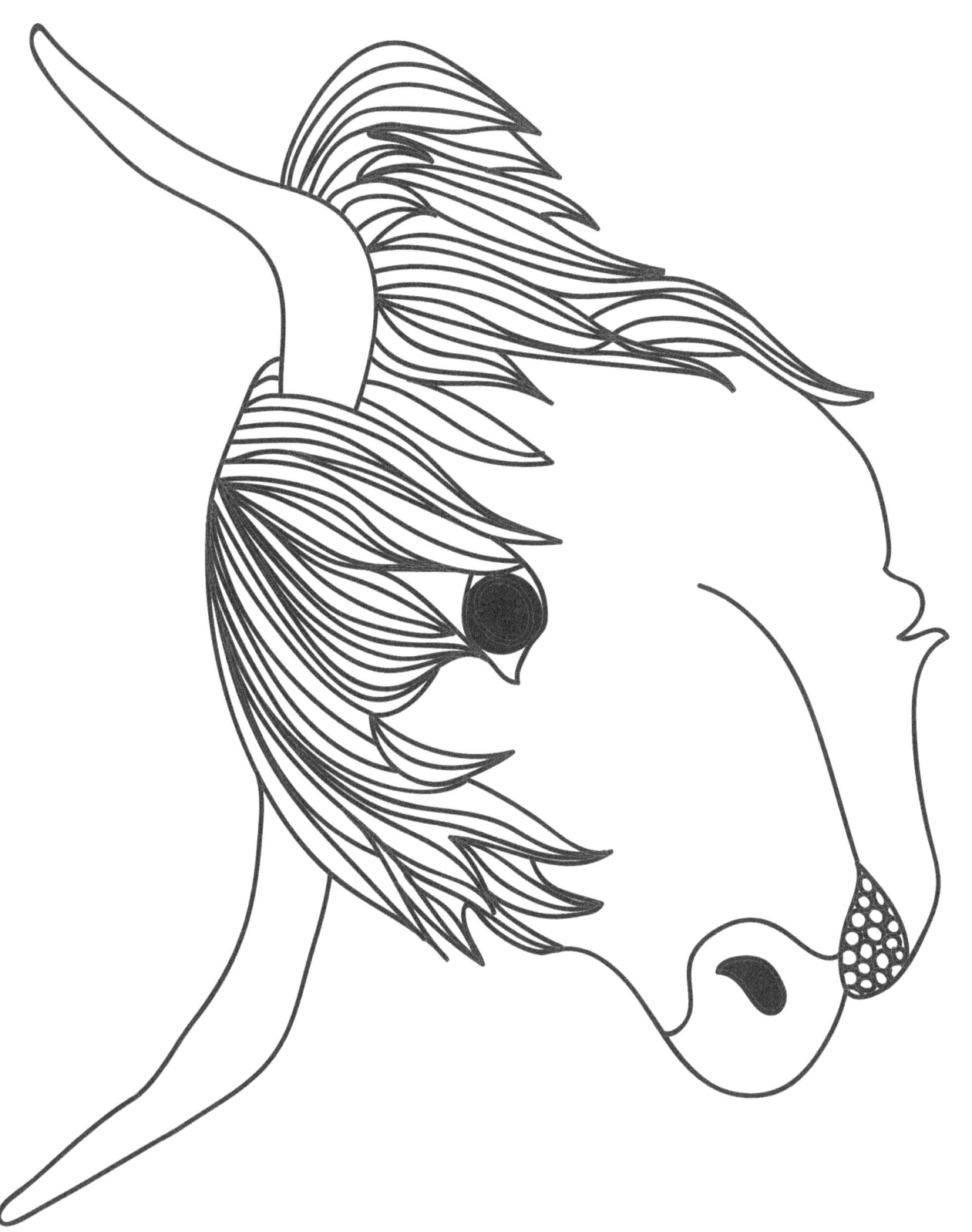

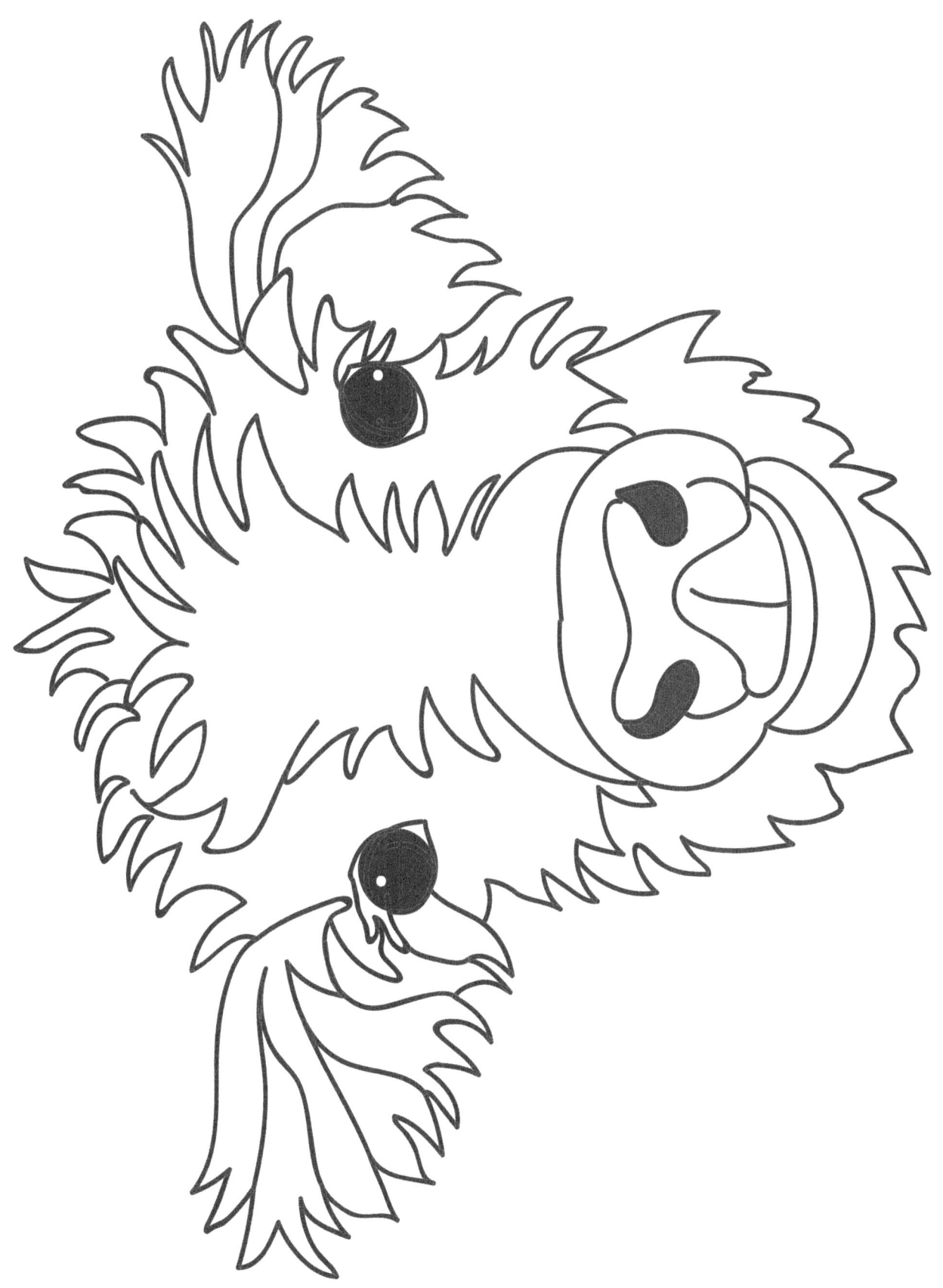

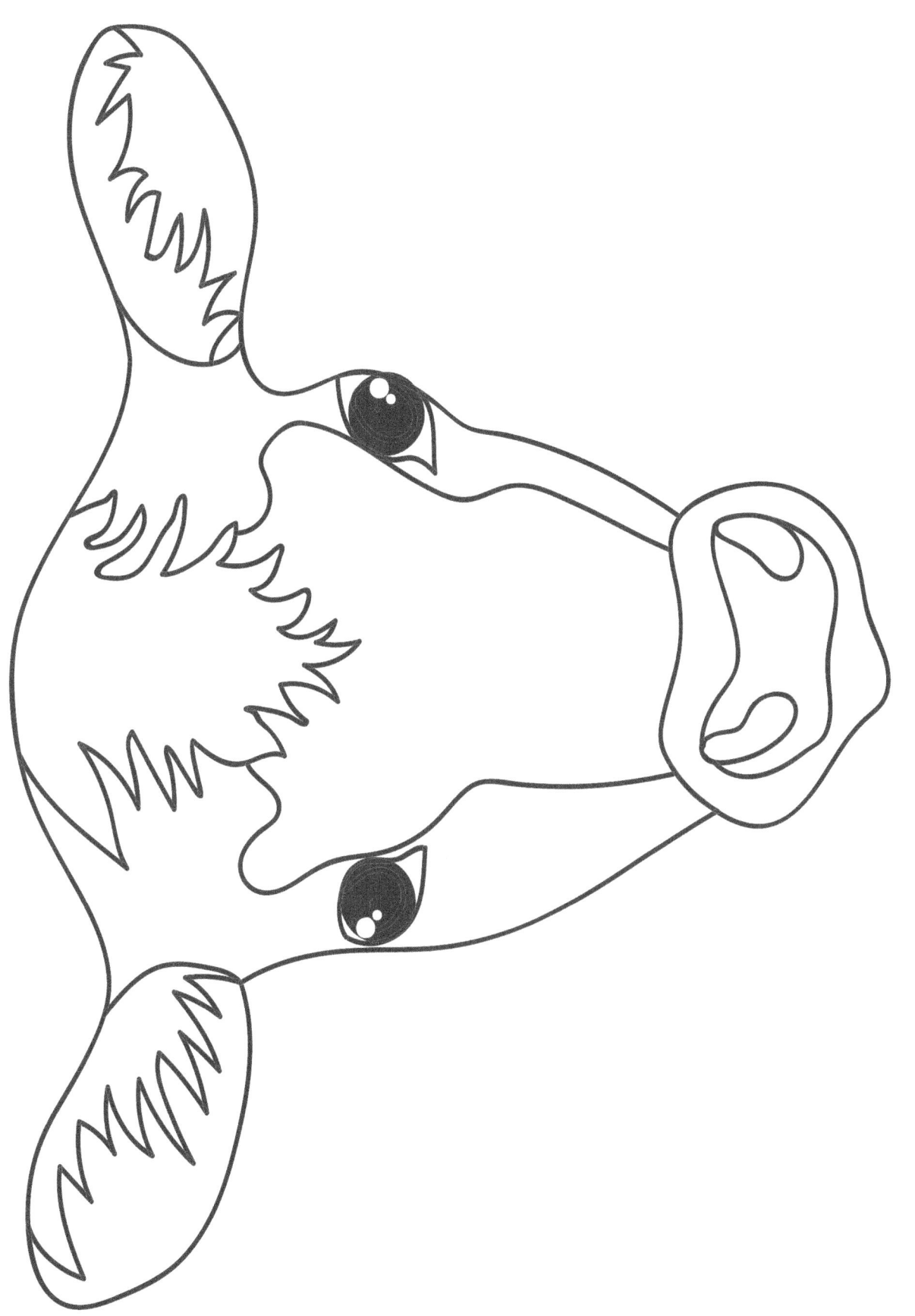

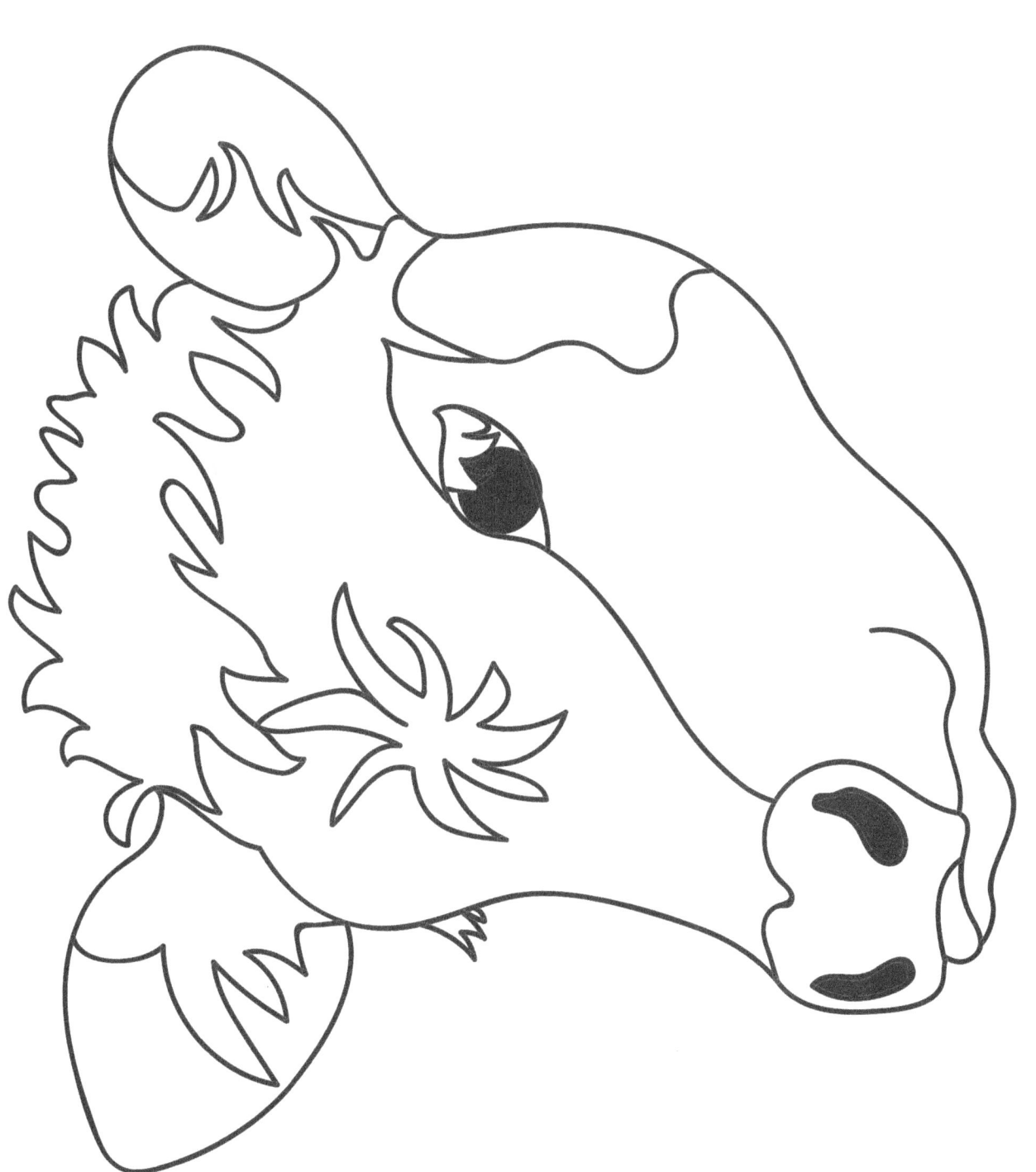

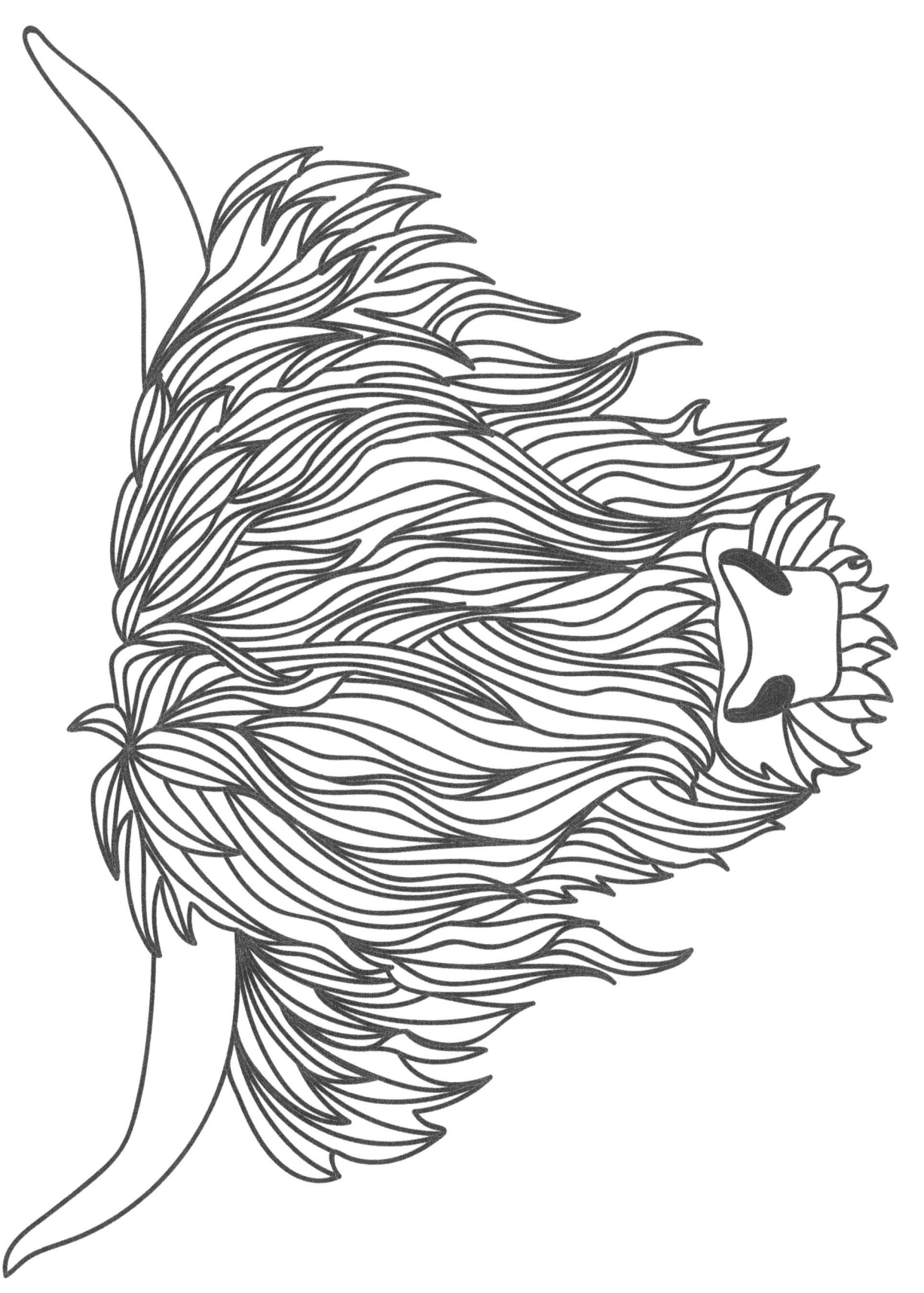

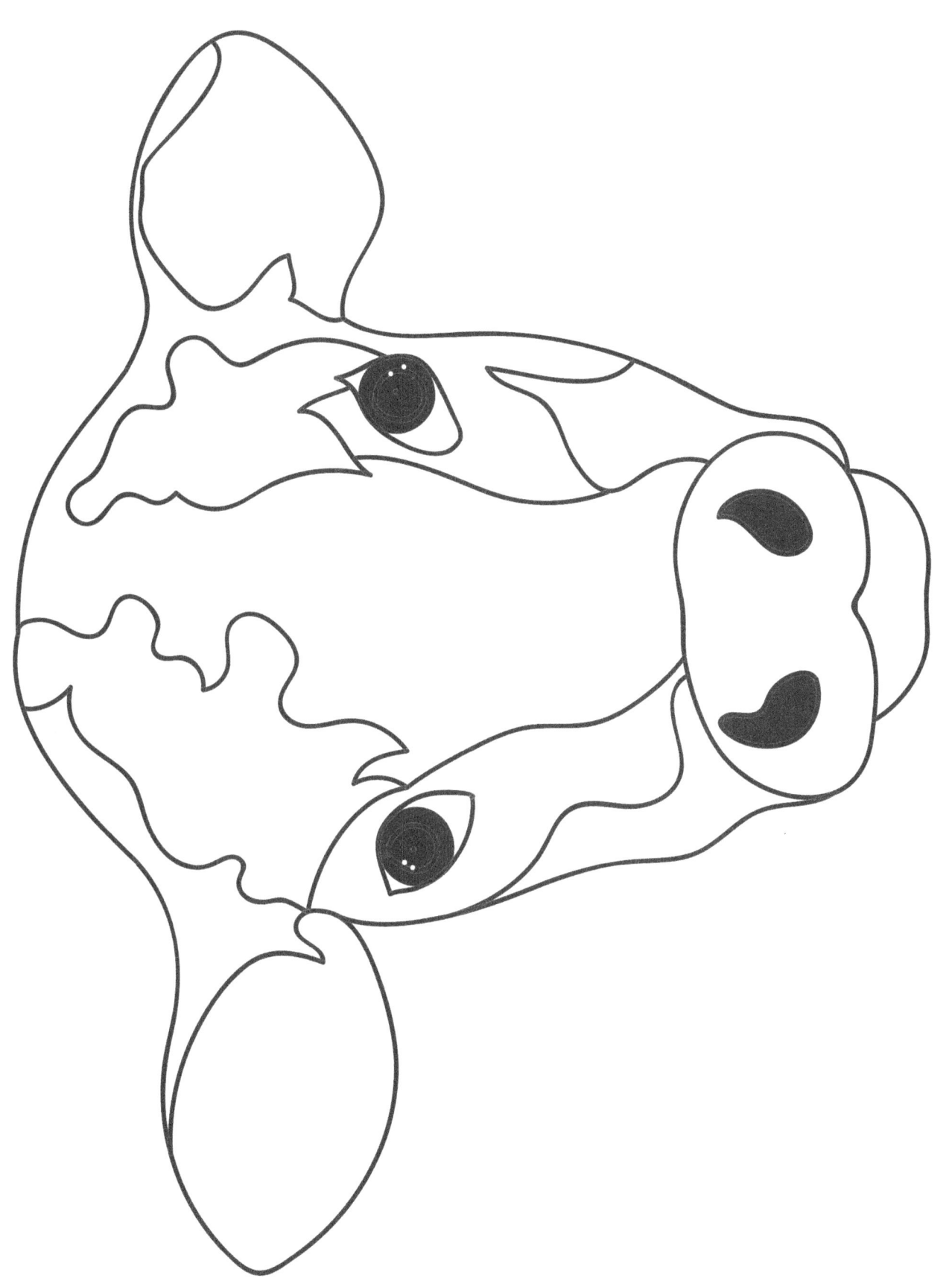

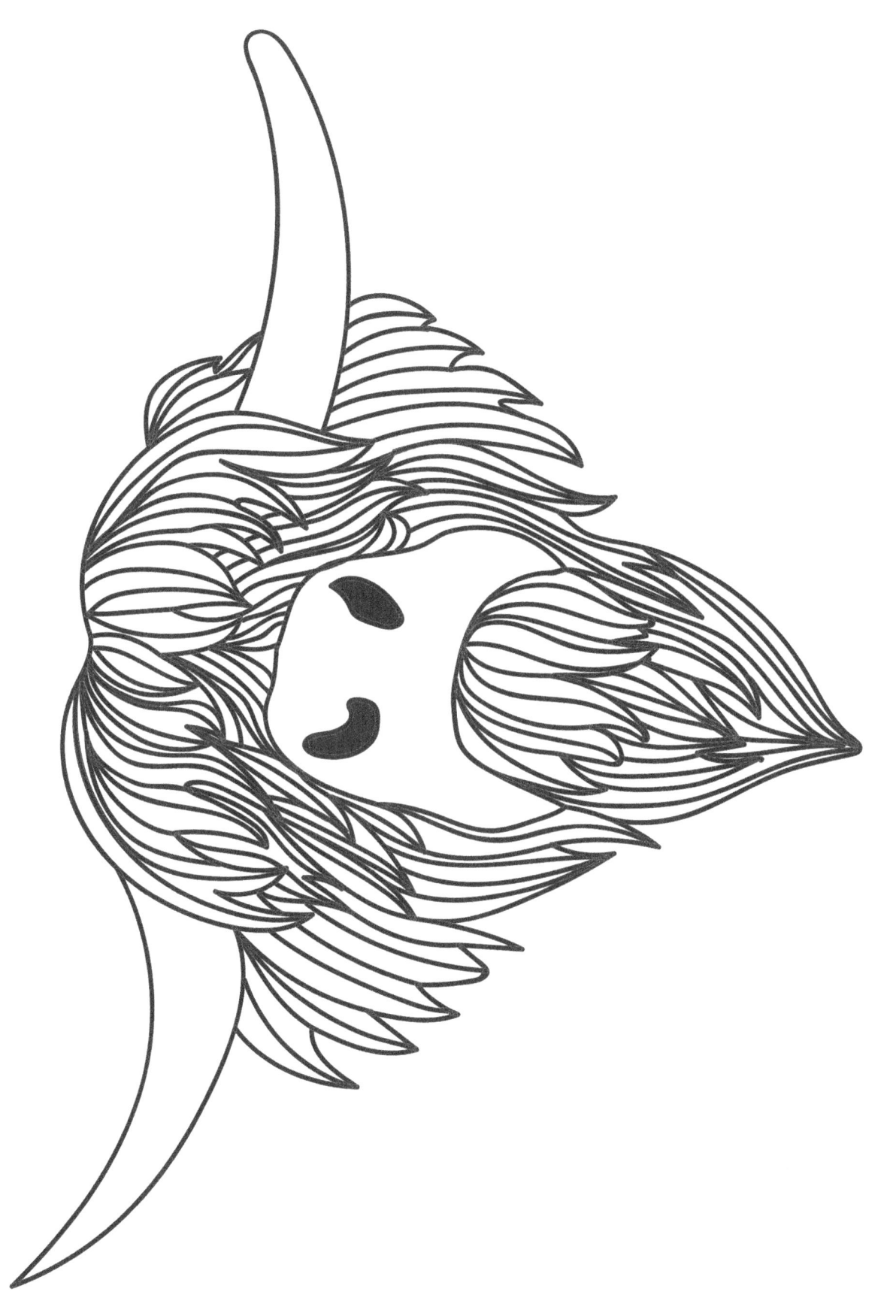

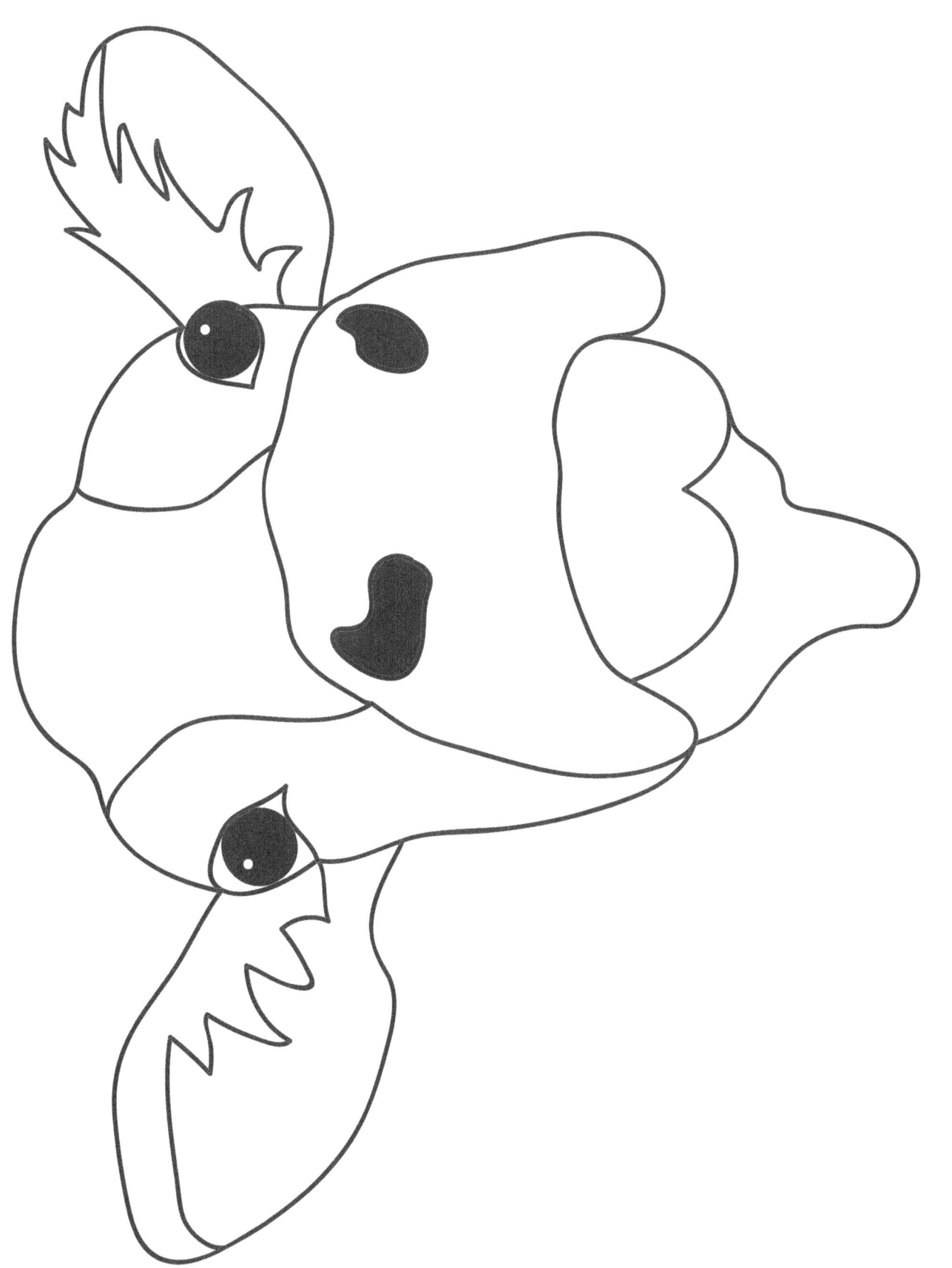

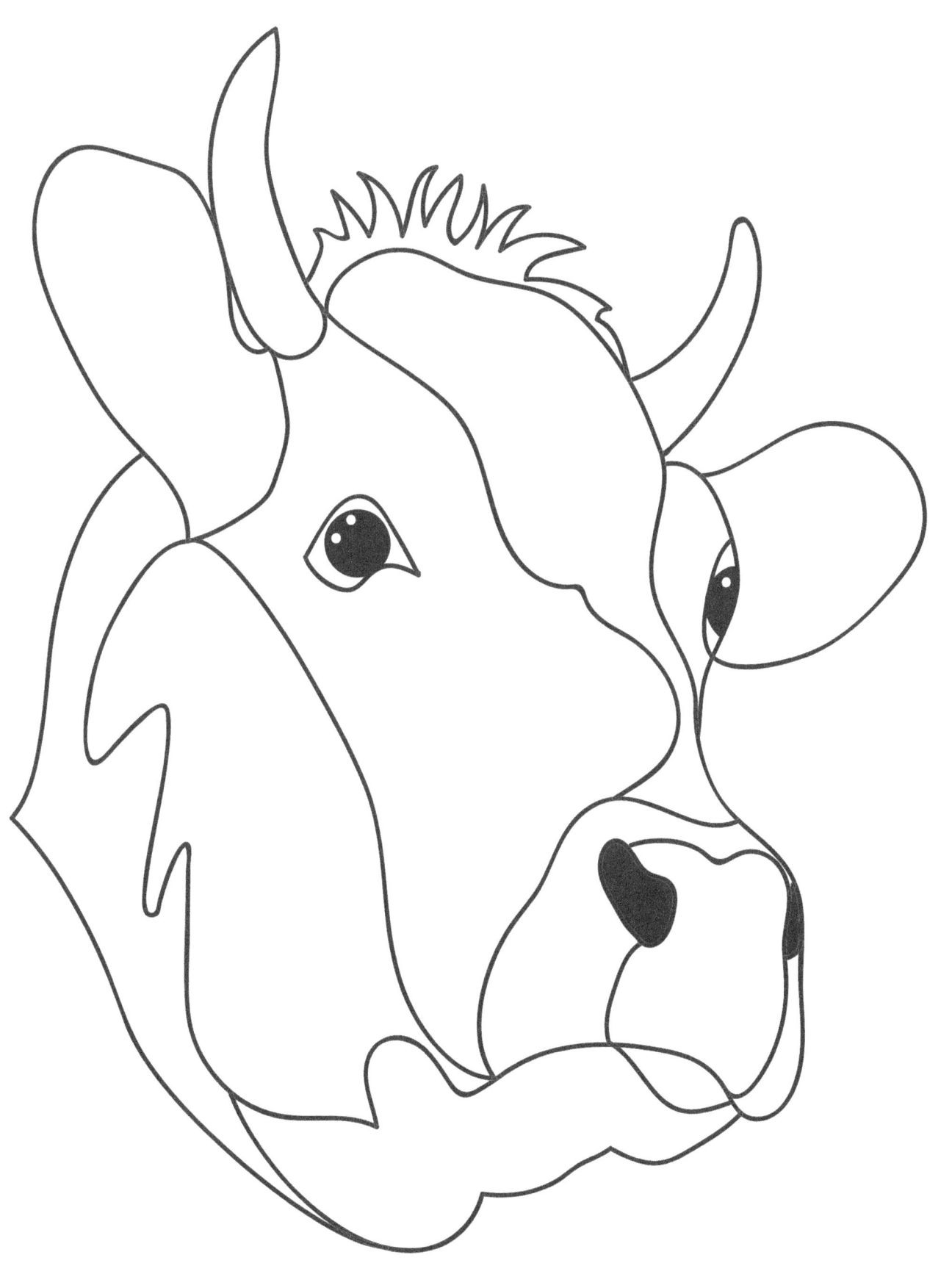

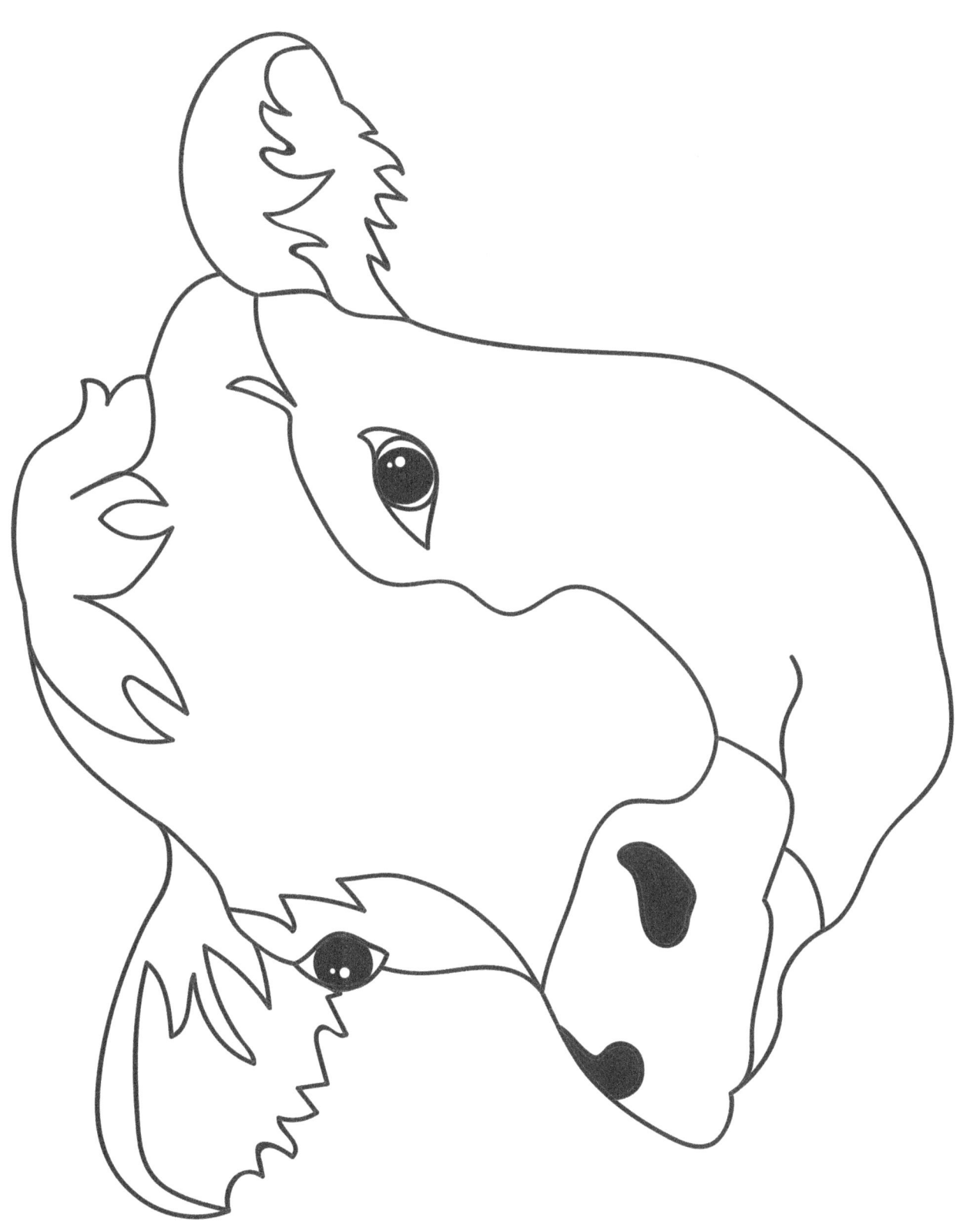

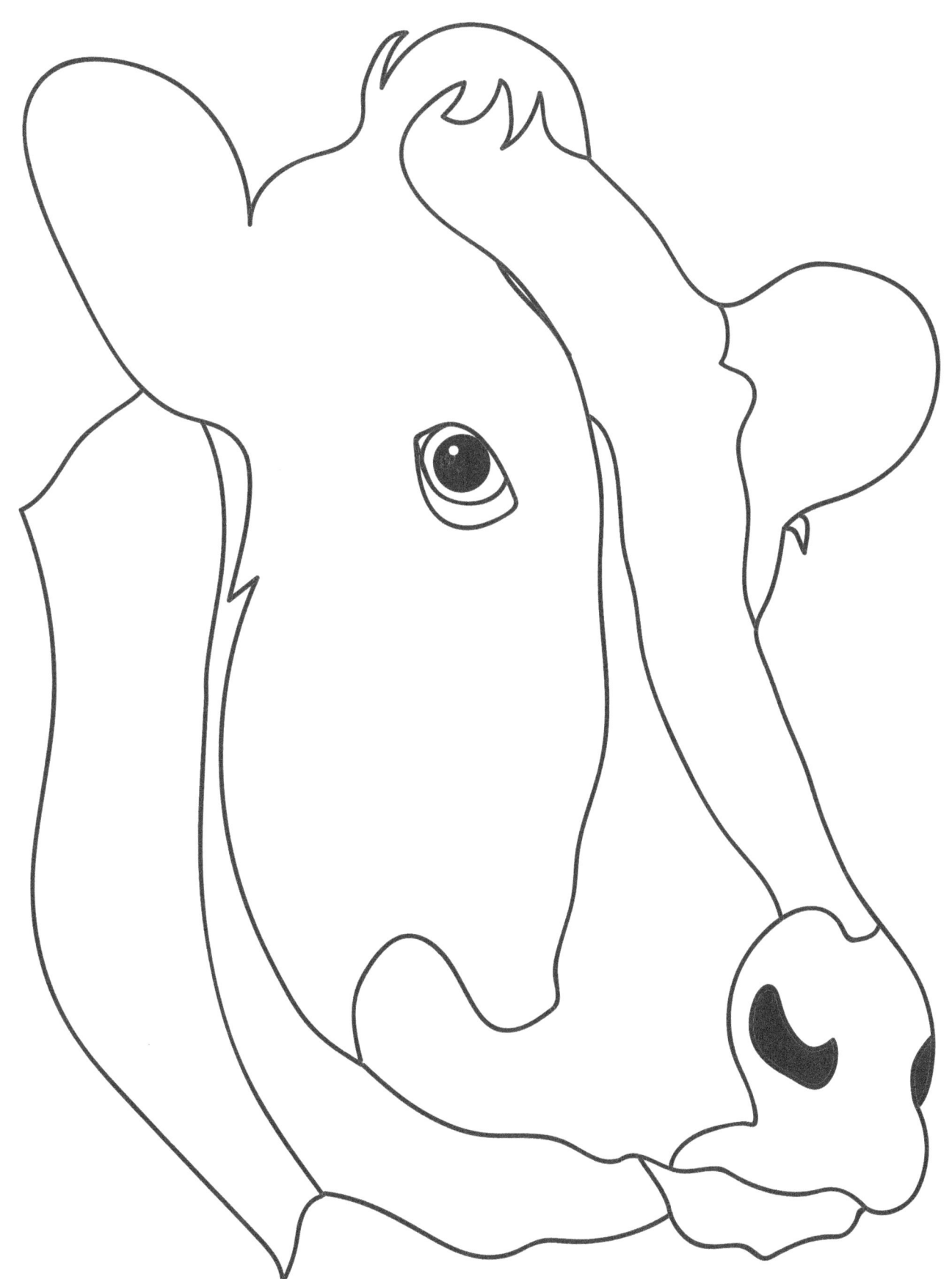

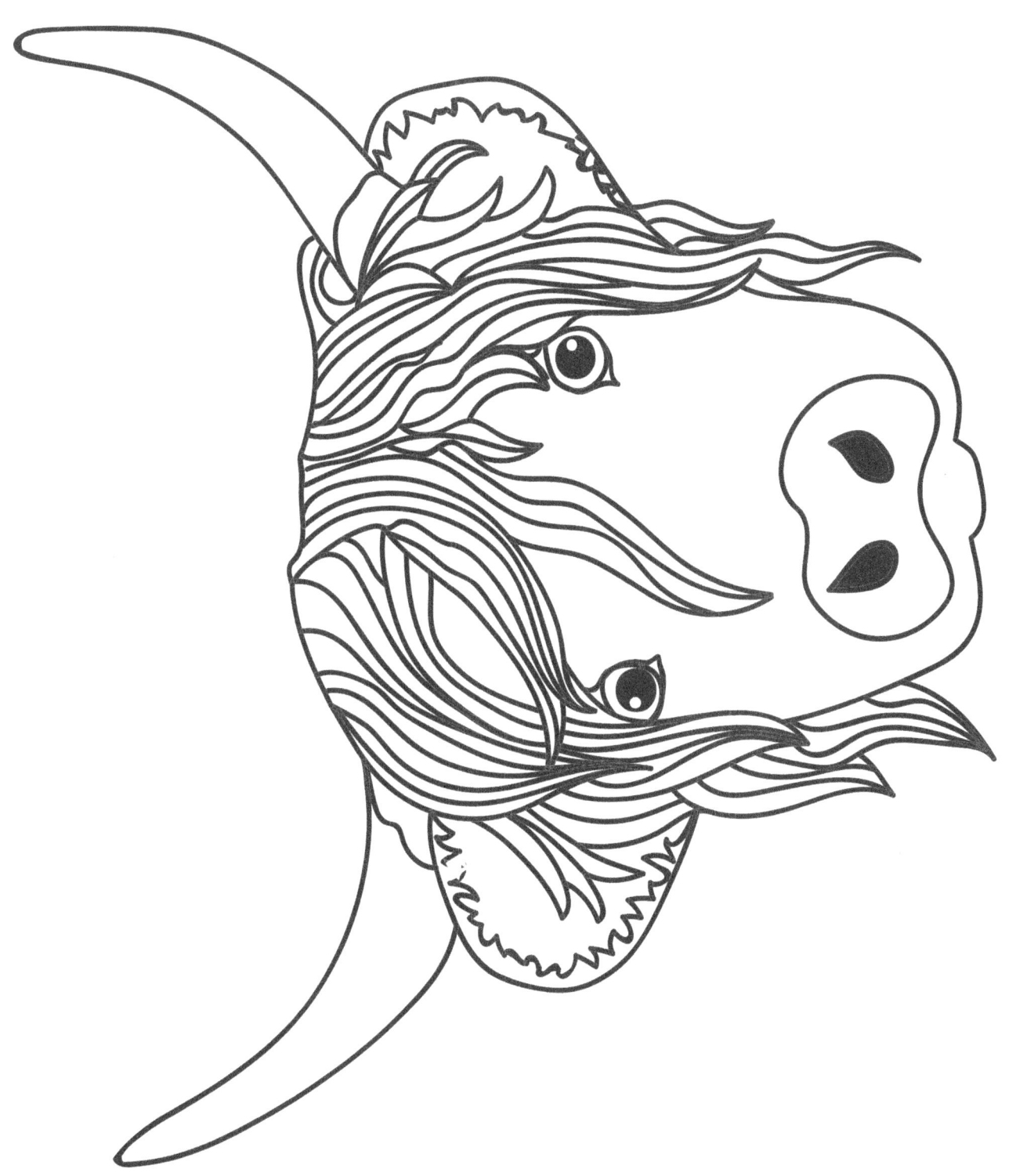

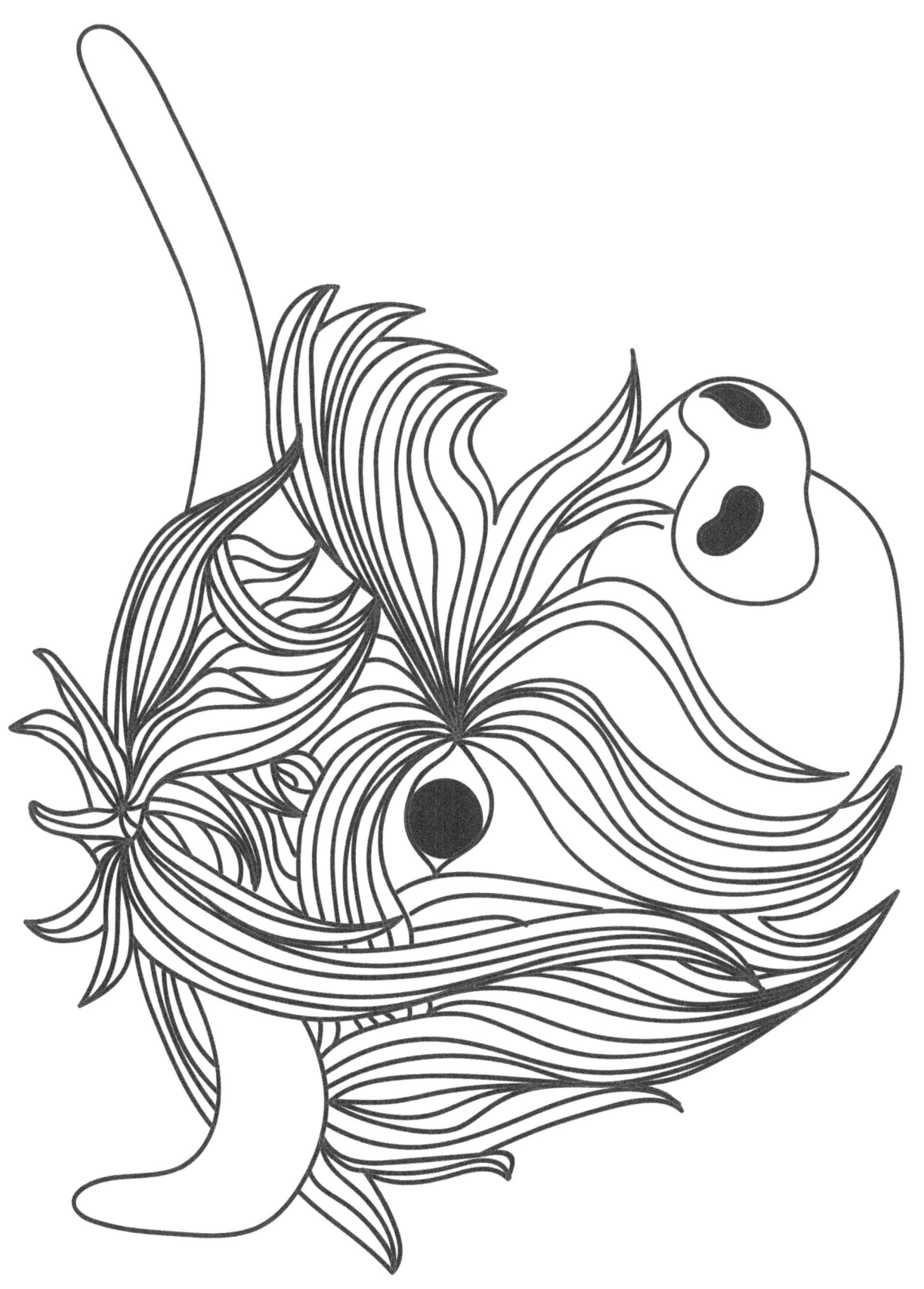

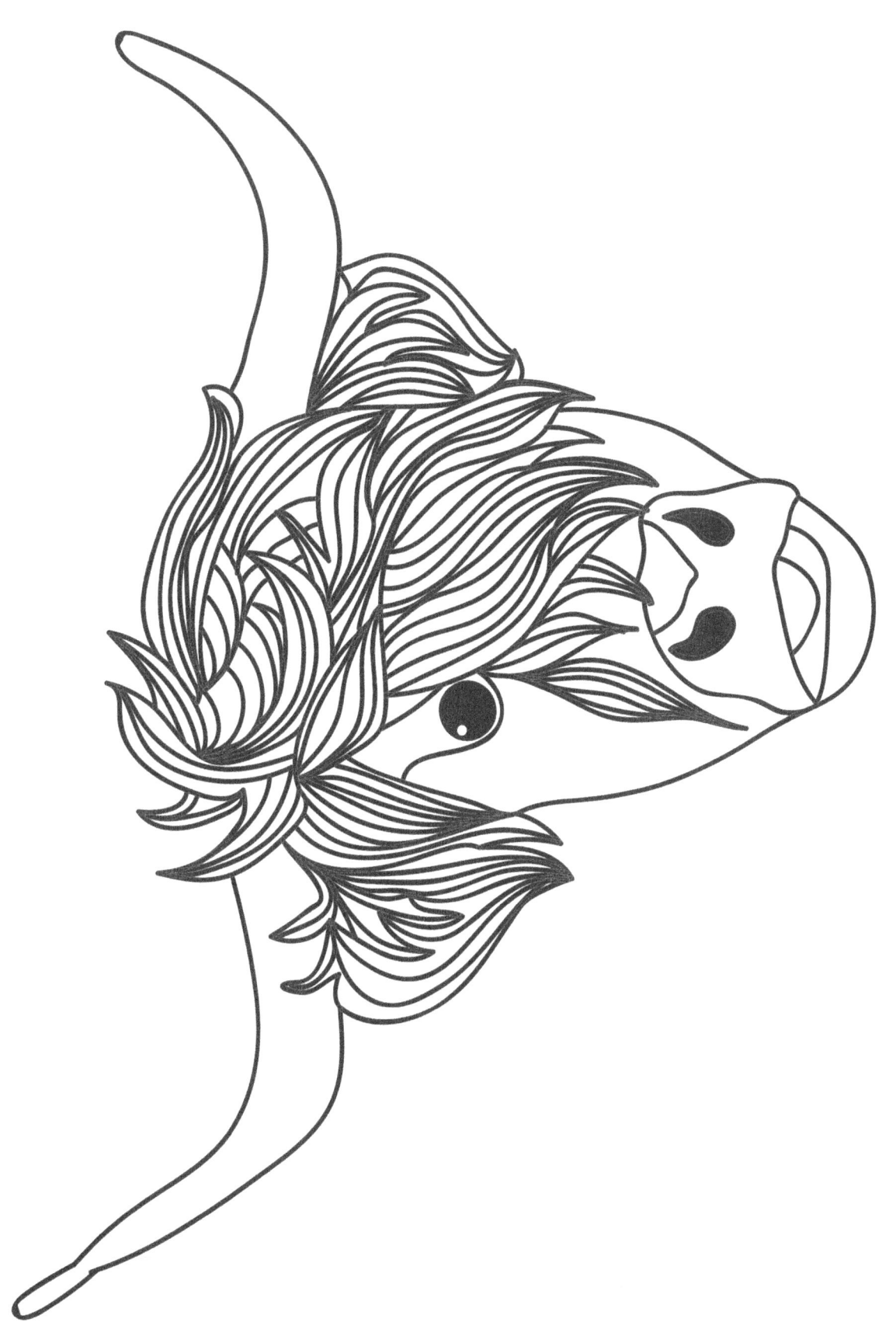

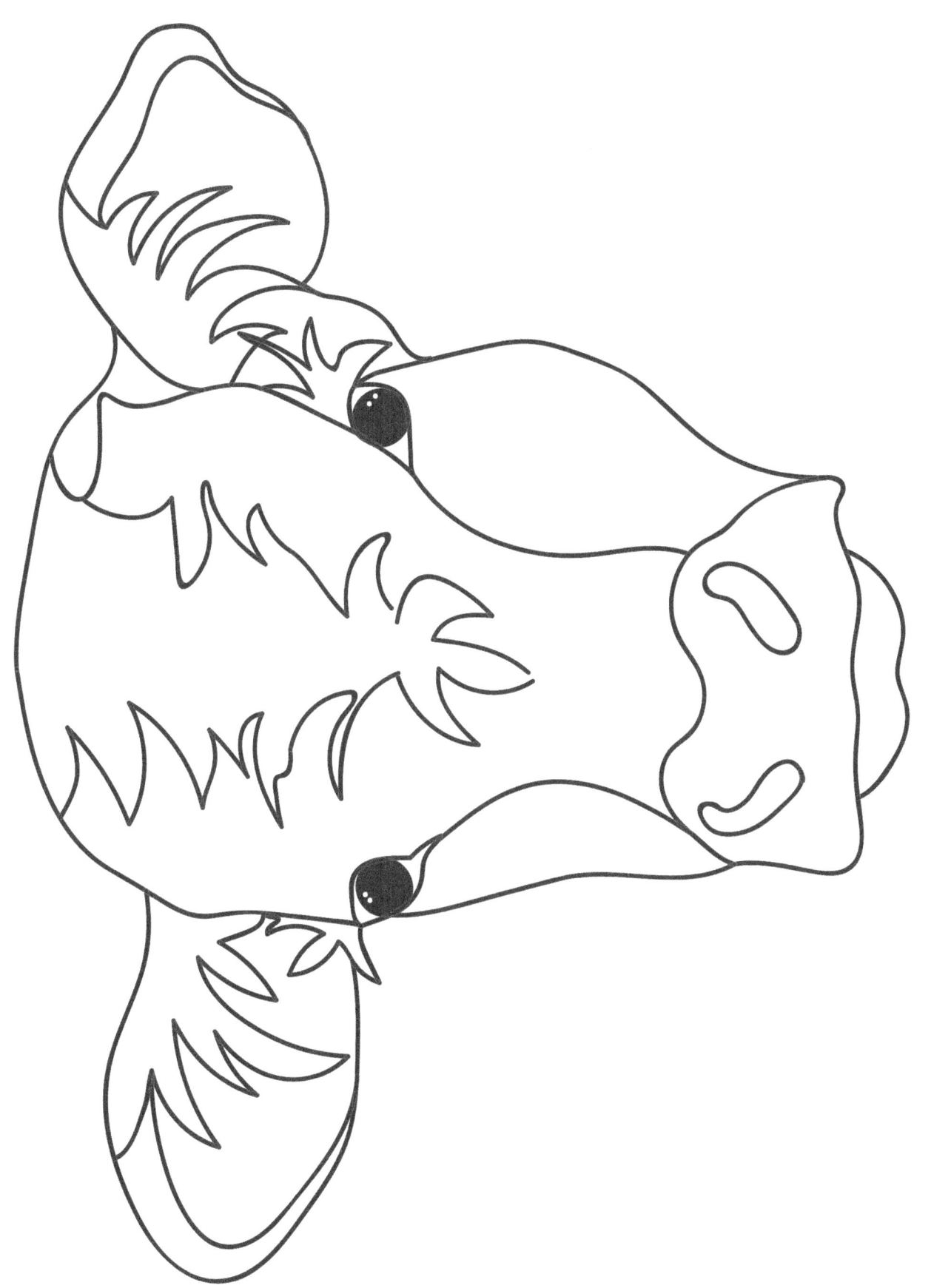

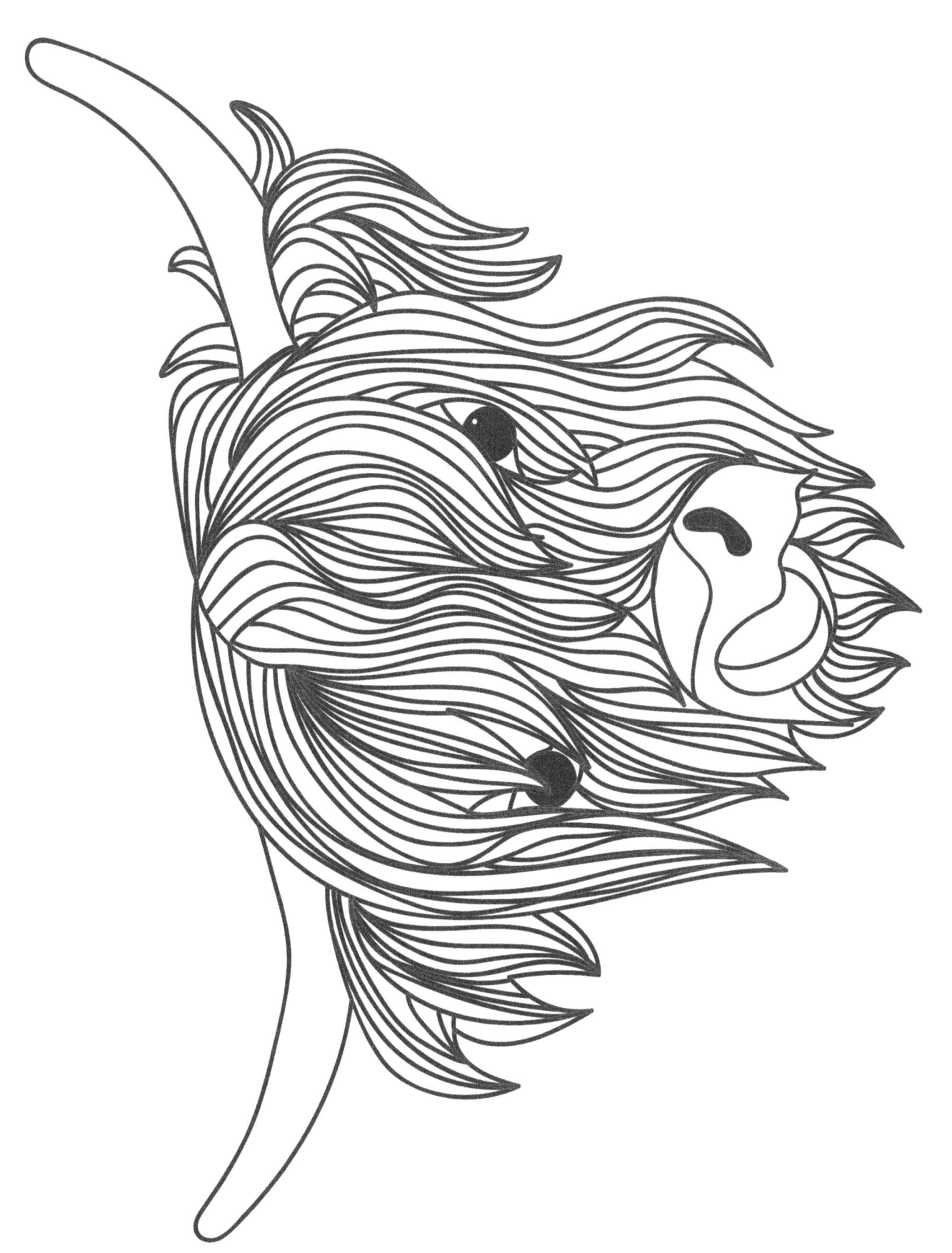

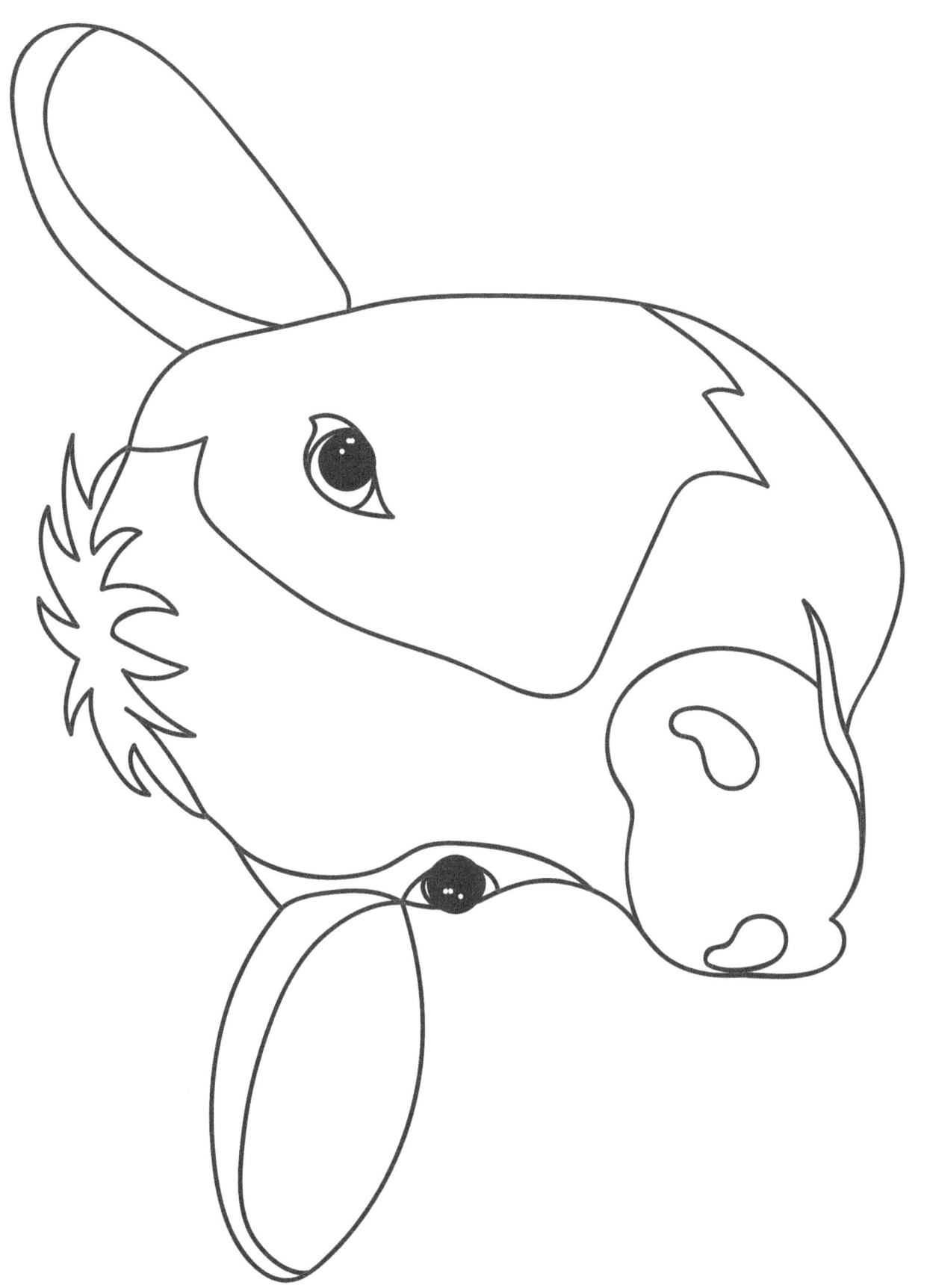

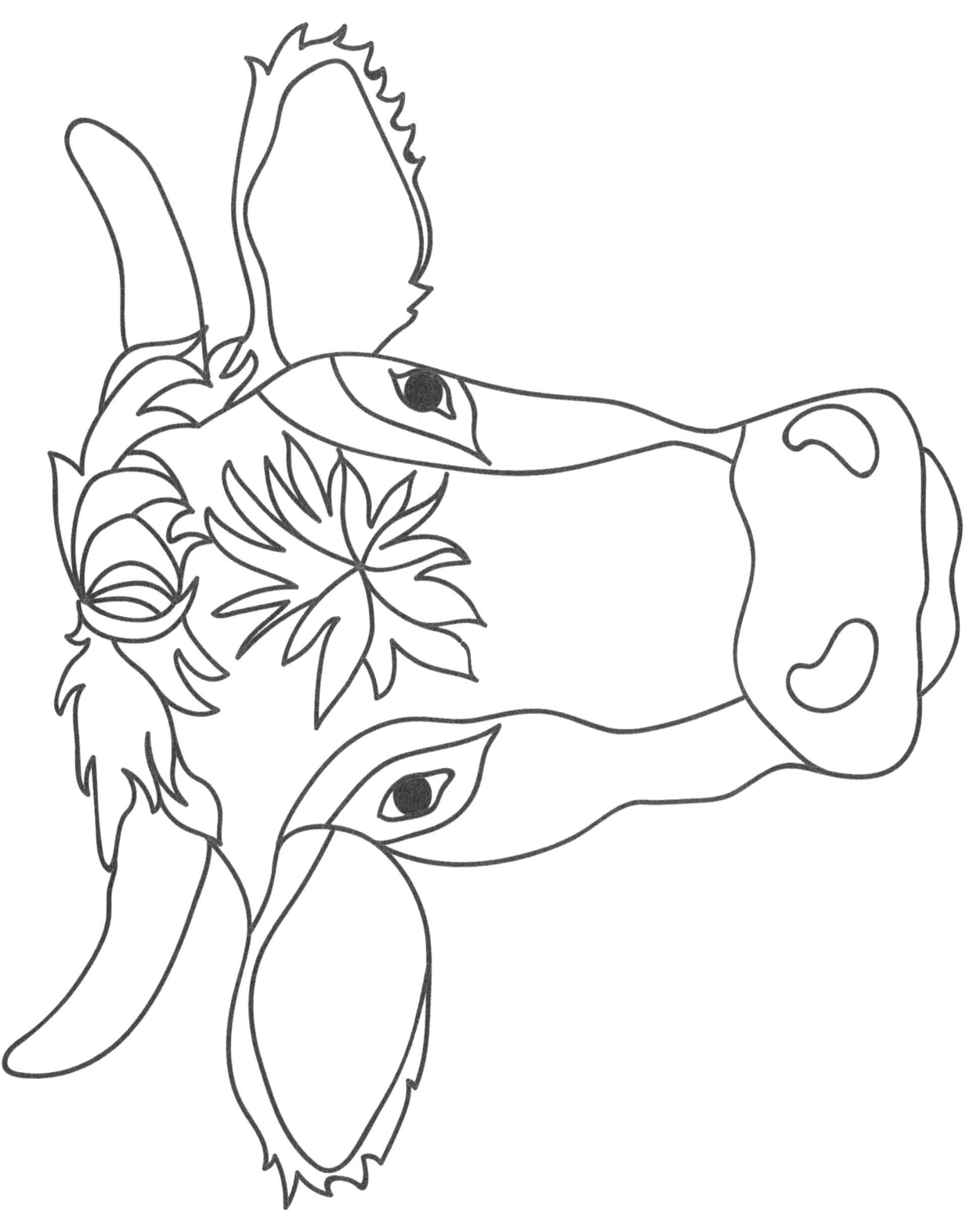

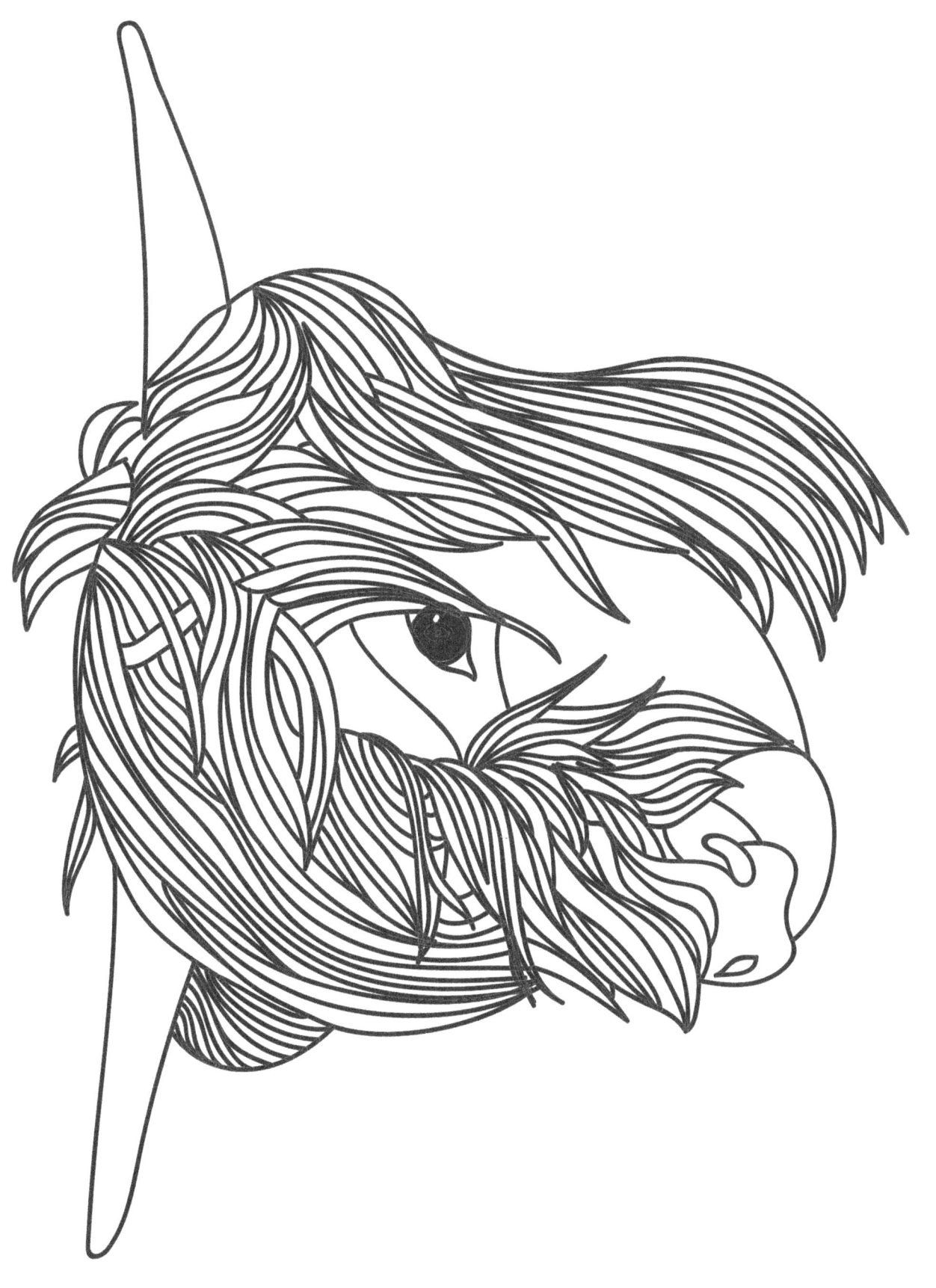

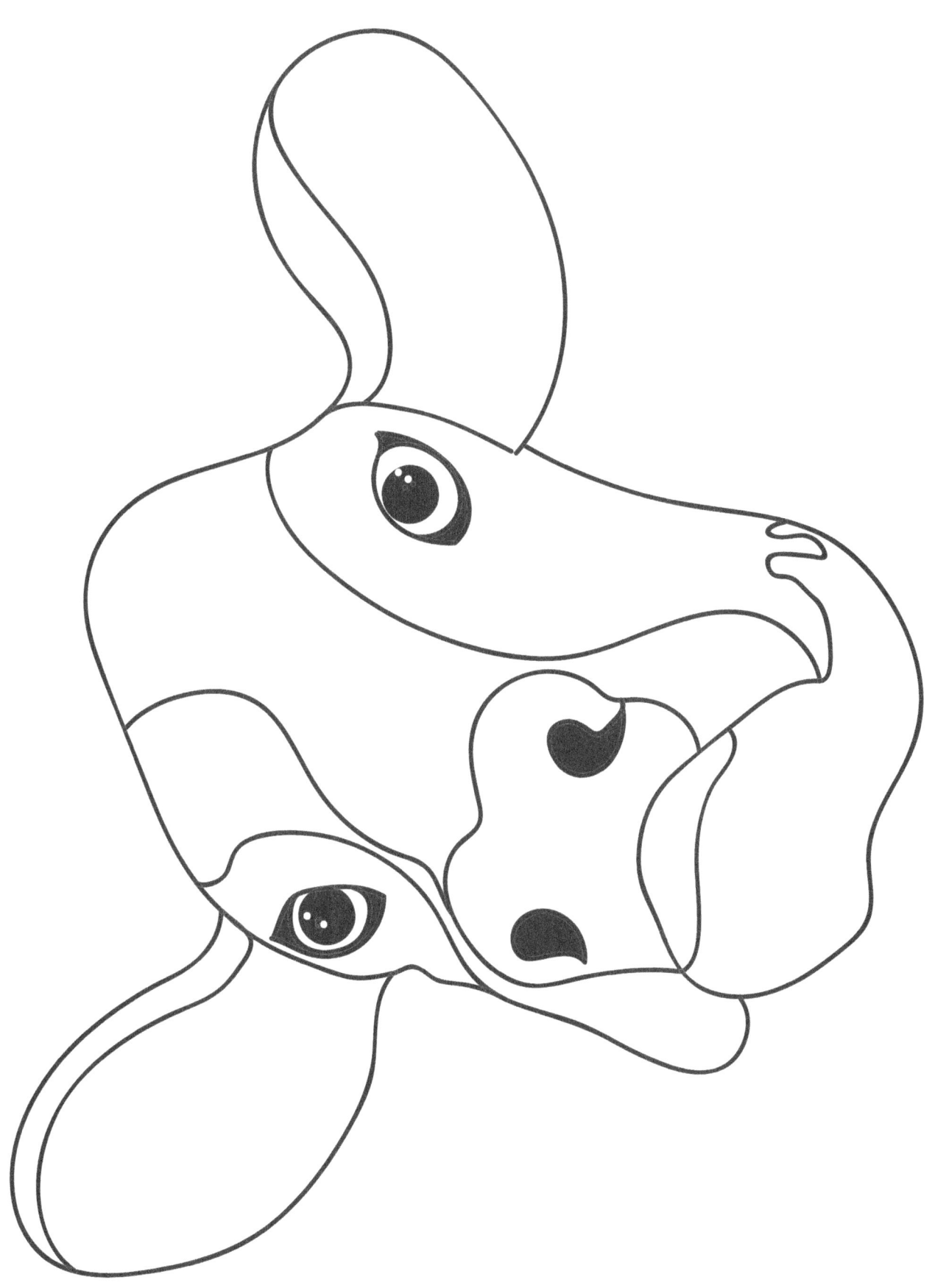

COLOR TEST PAGE

COLOR TEST PAGE

www.ingramcontent.com/pod-product-compliance
Lightning Source LLC
Chambersburg PA
CBHW062229220526
45471CB00009B/3408